Healing
with Copper

Healing
with Copper

THE COMPLETE GUIDE TO
ALLEVIATING FATIGUE,
BOOSTING **BRAIN FUNCTION,** AND
STRENGTHENING YOUR **IMMUNE SYSTEM**
WITH ESSENTIAL METALS

YVELETTE STINES

Published by:
ULYSSES PRESS
PO Box 3440
Berkeley, CA 94703
www.ulyssespress.com

ISBN: 978-1-64604-449-8
Library of Congress Control Number: 2022944064

Printed in the United States by Kingery Printing Company
10 9 8 7 6 5 4 3 2 1

Acquisitions editor: Casie Vogel
Project editor: Shelona Belfon
Managing editor: Claire Chun
Editor: Renee Rutledge
Proofreader: Joyce Wu
Front cover design: Hannah Pelz
Interior design and layout: Winnie Liu
Front and back cover art: shutterstock.com © Sadovnikova Olga

This book is dedicated to the people who are working hard to make their dreams come true.

Contents

Introduction

Take great care of yourself. You have one body and one life.

It is important that we take care of our health. This includes our physical health, mental health, and overall wellness. You've likely heard this many times over that you have to do the right things to keep your body and mind healthy. This includes eating nutritious foods, exercising, keeping stress levels low, getting enough rest, taking vitamins and minerals as needed, going to the doctor and/or mental health professional when required, and more.

Although these are general tips, there is no one-size-fits-all for creating and maintaining optimal health. Everyone has a different body type and genetic makeup, so what one person can do for their health can be completely different for the next person. It is important to understand that our health journey is ours and we should be patient with ourselves.

There are various ways to get healthy. Along with practicing healthy habits, you can educate yourself by taking a class, reading materials that can help you incorporate some of the information that you learned, or watching a lecture. If the new things that you learn are aligned with your lifestyle, try to incorporate some of the information. This can also help you decide whether the new habit or dietary regimen is something that you would like to continue.

If the information doesn't apply at the moment, pay it forward and share what you learned with someone else, or consider using the information for a different time in your life. Sometimes it takes listening to or reading the information more than once to truly process and understand where and how the information can fit into your life. We all have different learning styles and preferences. Embrace yours and enjoy the process of learning.

This book is about the health and healing benefits of copper. While minerals can serve multiple purposes, copper affects many areas of our lives. Copper was the first metal to be used by humans, serving as a material for tools, weapons, and crafts throughout history, and it is still very relevant today. From the time the sun rises in the morning to the time it sets, most of us have some direct or indirect involvement with copper.

Imagine this: the sun is glowing through the window and your alarm starts to notify you that it is time to wake up. As you reach for your cell phone or clock (yes, those still exist) to turn off the alarm, copper is involved. If you're using an alarm clock, its circuit board includes elements of copper. As you get out of bed, making your way to the bathroom to brush your teeth and shower, copper is involved. There are traces of copper in the tap water due to the corrosion of the plumbing that is made from copper. In addition, copper is a natural mineral found in lakes and rivers. From washing your face to using certain personal-care products like lotion and cosmetics, copper is involved.

As you get dressed, if you use certain jewelry, clothing, and accessories, you guessed it: copper is involved. From eating breakfast like avocado toast or Greek yogurt to leaving for your morning commute, copper has its place, as subways, cars, and buses all have elements of copper. Even if you work from home, there are elements of copper involved. As the day ends and you cook and eat dinner, from the appliances that are used, some dishes, and certain kitchen items, copper is involved. Finally, we can't forget the beloved penny. If you are making a purchase and using cash (yes, we still do that too) and you need those one or two cents, a small percent of copper is involved.

As you can see, copper is deeply ingrained in our world. Another area where copper is necessary and affects daily life is health and healing. High levels of copper is not necessary to sustain health. If you eat foods that have enough copper, it is not too difficult to meet the daily requirement. Having proper amounts of copper in the body can help it function properly and stay healthy.

One of copper's many roles is sustaining the health of the immune system, connective tissue, and red blood cells. Copper also aids in forming collagen and reducing free radicals in the body.

Certain illnesses, such as celiac disease, inflammatory bowel disease, Crohn's disease, and Menkes disease, can cause a copper deficiency, as can undergoing some surgeries, such as gastric bypass surgery. A deficiency of copper in the diet can lead to a number of health conditions such as osteoporosis and anemia. There are other conditions that will be discussed in Chapter Three.

The body doesn't produce copper on its own, so it's important to get it through food. I know it doesn't seem very appetizing to think of consuming copper, but don't worry, many wonderful and delicious foods contain it. (We'll go over these foods in greater detail in Chapter Seven, Food and Copper.) You can also get copper through supplements, which I'll cover in Chapter Eight.

As with all vitamins and minerals, it is important to know your levels to ensure you have the proper amounts to stay healthy and your body can function properly. Your vitamin levels can be measured through a blood test given by your doctor or an at-home vitamin deficiency kit.

What You Can Expect from This Book

In the pages of this book, you will learn more about the specific ways that copper can heal the body and support optimal health. You will learn about the ways copper can improve your immune system, help brain function, increase energy, and relieve symptoms of chronic illness. In addition, I will share some steps that you can take to properly incorporate copper into your diet.

The choices that you make in the present moment will impact you years down the line. Remember, before starting any new exercise or incorporating new foods and vitamins, consult your doctor. They can help you determine the right plan for your lifestyle.

Learning a new skill or habit takes time. The steps you take along the way create the difference. Whether it is exercising, creating new recipes for healthier eating, or reading new material to improve any area of your life, focus on the small steps to mastery.

In addition to serving as your introductory guide to copper as a healing mineral, this book will also include general information on health practices to help you understand the bigger picture. Read this book at your leisure or use it as a resource if you want to refresh your knowledge on some of the ways copper serves as a healing property.

When it comes to overall wellness, be kind to yourself and others. Each day, do something that your future self will thank you for. Again, small steps in the right direction can lead to life-changing results. As you step toward a healthier you, mind, body, and soul, take notes and photos of your process, how you felt, and the improvements that you made along the way, so you will have a beautiful recollection to see how far you've come. Each day won't be perfect, but document the imperfect days by writing down what you did to cope with any struggles that came up. This exercise is another way that you can get to know yourself and the way you move through adversity. It's all too easy to focus on the outward aspects of growth, but the internal is just as important.

I hope this book encourages you to take aligned and healthy steps toward living a life that you love. I hope the information it contains is digestible and impactful enough for you to understand the importance of copper and the impact that it has on your health.

Happy reading!

CHAPTER ONE

A Holistic Approach to Health

Before we delve into the specific ways that copper can benefit your body, this chapter will focus on setting goals for creating a healthy lifestyle from a holistic perspective.

If you want to improve or change any area in your life, you have to start from the inside. It takes awareness, determination, focus, and consistent action to create and sustain a healthy life. When you take a holistic approach to well-being, you reflect and recognize the areas that are working well, the areas where you can use some tweaks for improvement, and the areas that need change. You will start to see how each area in your life will affect other areas. You will become more conscious and take the steps to become a better version of yourself. Once you identify the specific areas in your life that you would like to improve, start with small intentional steps to do the work that you need to do to create a life that you love.

Make the Decision to Live a Life You Love

If we don't have our health, we can't have the fulfilling life that we deserve. This goes beyond just physical health but encompasses our emotional, environmental, financial, intellectual, social, and spiritual health as well. There are times when some areas are wonderful and others could use some fine-tuning. That is why it is important to take the time you need to reflect and assess where you are and where you would like to be. Being honest with ourselves and understanding who we are, where we are in life, who we want to become, and where we are going takes time and effort. It also takes a lot of self-awareness, reflection, patience, and truly understanding ourselves. As with any relationship, give yourself time, grace, and understanding. Your thoughts and behaviors make a big difference in how you show up in the world. The change starts with your mind and then taking consistent action. Set an intention and make a clear decision on the areas that you would like to change in your life..

Change can come with some resistance due to hanging on to familiarity. Some may fear the unknown. Change creates growth and beautiful experiences. Rightfully so, it can be scary to charter into unknown waters. As you make the effort to change, having a support system is very helpful and for some, it is necessary. Whether it is a class, coach, therapist, or accountability partner, a support system can help you grow into a new version of yourself.

With the willingness, determination, and consistency that you commit to, a favorable change is inevitable. Taking it step by step, you will get closer to achieving your goals and seeing the change that you want to make in your world. There will be challenges along the way, and some of the challenges that you encounter are inevitable. Take the lessons you've learned and apply the knowledge to help you grow even more. In the face of adversity, take your time, get the help that you need, pause when you need to, and continue toward the positive path that you are creating.

Are You Taking Care of Yourself?

Are you taking care of yourself to the best of your ability? If your answer is yes, wonderful! Continue and improve from where you are. If your answer is no, today is a wonderful day to start taking the necessary steps to take better care of yourself. Now, if your self-care has not been a high priority, you are not alone. Many of us are so busy meeting the demands of our to-do list that it seems to grow more and more each day, and somehow, we end up at the bottom of the list or not on the list at all. Time moves so quickly, we are not aware that we missed the mark on taking care of ourselves. So, if you had to pause and think about the question and realized that you don't take great care of yourself, give yourself a compassionate hug for acknowledging your truth. The self-awareness and acknowledgment is a beautiful start.

Congratulations, you now have the awareness that you would like to take better care of yourself!

The next step is reflection. Take some time to think about the areas you want to improve in your life. Think about the part you play now and how you would like to show up in specific areas of your life. Write those areas down. Don't overthink the process of writing, just make a bulleted list of items that come to mind. You can organize it later.

Once you complete your list, categorize each goal into a specific category. For this exercise, we will use the seven categories from the Wellness Wheel, a concept developed by Dr. Bill Hettler, cofounder of the National Wellness Institute. The categories of the Wellness Wheel are interconnected, together contributing to overall well-being. They are emotional, environmental, financial, intellectual, physical, social, and spiritual. According to the National Wellness Institute, The Wellness Wheel can bring awareness to the following areas of your life:

o A healthy sense of self-esteem, determination, a sense of purpose, and clear direction.

o Building and sustaining a healthy living space.

o Creating healthy relationships and social networks.

o Creating and sustaining habits of healthy living, such as self-care, exercise, personal responsibility, eating habits, and maintaining a healthy lifestyle.

o Enjoying others within and outside of your community.

o Life balance and enrichment through work, socialization, continued education, and enjoyment.

o Making contributions to the community and/or organizations that are important to you.

o Utilizing your gifts and engaging in creative and intellectually stimulating activities.

o Understanding and living aligned with your development of values and belief systems.

Below I delve into each category of the Wellness Wheel in greater detail:

Emotional—This category encourages you to address your emotional state. It invites you to evaluate the ways that you acknowledge and address your feelings. As you move through your world, reflect on your actions when it comes to the ways that you handle disappointment, overcome challenges, and navigate stressful situations. This is a space where you can also reflect on your wins and the positive things that are happening in your life. Are you open to sharing and celebrating yourself or do you shy away from bringing attention to your wins? The emotional category also encourages you to explore how you interact with yourself and your relationships.

Environmental—This category covers the environment and spaces that you engage in on a regular basis. Examine the areas in which you spend a lot of time. Think about how you feel. Pay attention to your breathing in these spaces. Do you feel calm or anxious?

Your environment has a strong impact on your mental and physical health. You may feel comfortable in a space without realizing it may be affecting your health. Think about the area where you spend the majority of your time. As you imagine the area, picture the whole space and reflect on the way you are breathing. The cleanliness, clutter, old items, corners, and where things are placed all have an effect on your health.

If there is a lot of clutter, consider cleaning it out. Clutter is known to create extra stress, cause a lack of focus, and affect your memory. There are situations and circumstances where a change of environment is not an option. Generally speaking, do the best you can with what you have. If you are in a situation where you feel unsafe in your environment, get the help that you need so you will be able to feel safe and healthy.

Financial—This category relates to your career, career goals, financial health, and responsibility. Think about the work that you do and the purpose behind it. If you are not doing the work that you want to do, think about what you can do to change that.

Examine and reflect on areas that you are passionate about and how you can pivot into doing the work that interests you. Reflect on your financial status, well-being, and attitude and beliefs about making, spending, and keeping money. Remember that your value as a human being and/or level of importance is not aligned with your profession or the amount of money that you make. As with any area in life, it is perfectly fine to hire someone to help you with your career goals and financial planning.

Intellectual—This category relates to your intellectual advancement and participation. Examine the intellectually stimulating activities that you participate in on a regular basis. Reflect and determine whether or not you feel and/or engage in activities that enhance your intellect.

Physical—This category relates to your physical health. Look at your habits when it comes to exercise, eating, staying hydrated, getting enough sleep, and adhering to your medical needs in a timely and appropriate manner. Try to understand the motivation and reasons behind your habits and actions when it comes to your physical health.

Social—The social category speaks to the quality of your interaction with others and the quality of your social life. Reflect on your personal involvement within your family, friends, community, coworkers, and society as a whole. Having healthy and supportive social interactions can help prevent feelings of loneliness, stress, and isolation.

Spiritual—Spiritual wellness is aligned with finding meaning and purpose in life. It also encourages you to look beyond yourself and seek a higher power of belief and faith. Many also align this category with their religious beliefs. Activities like prayer, meditation, and worship are activities that can be practiced with spiritual wellness.[1]

Once you are done with the bulleted list of areas you would like to improve in your life, categorize each of the items into one of the seven sections of the Wellness Wheel, and pick one or two goals for the month to start. If you are feeling extra motivated, pick more goals for the month. You can also take note of some areas that are working well and that you would like to continue. This can be a goal as well.

For example, if you started cooking more at home instead of going out to eat, make it a goal to continue and sustain that habit. You can add to the habit and learn four new recipes for the month. This covers your intellectual, physical, and financial areas. You are learning something new, eating healthy, and saving money by cooking at home. If you want to invite friends over to try your new recipe, you have now covered the social section of the Wellness Wheel.

Once you have written your goal(s), set the date that you want to complete the goal and write down the steps you need to take to complete each specific goal. Some goals can take five minutes

---

1 "Six Dimensions of Wellness—National Wellness Institute," *National Wellness Institute*, 2022, https://nationalwellness.org/resources/six -dimensions-of-wellness.

and others will take longer. It all depends. Give yourself dead-lines along the way. It is also useful to have an accountably partner to help you stay on track.

You can repeat this exercise to set new goals. Depending on where you are and the capacity that you have, start small. If you want to challenge yourself, add more goals. If you are already on track, keep going.

Don't Overthink It. Just Get Started.

Sometimes starting a new habit can be overwhelming. Many people start to overthink the goal. This can lead to telling ourselves a lot of excuses as to why we can't get started. Remember, anyone who is a master in a specific area started as a beginner. Here are some ideas for getting started.

o If you want to start exercising and you haven't gotten off the couch, start by walking 30 minutes a day.

o If you want to meditate and don't know how, get an app and do a 10-day meditation challenge by yourself or with some friends.

o If you want to get more fit, hire a trainer and nutritionist. If a trainer or nutritionist is not an option, start by reading books and implementing what you learn. You can find some great workouts on YouTube. Begin there and refine your goals as you progress.

o If you want to improve your nutritional health, set a goal to drink two more glasses of water a day and/or eliminate one unhealthy item from your diet.

o If you want to meet people or find a new hobby, take a class that looks interesting. Volunteer or find community activities that interest you.

o If you want to learn more about a topic, read books about the topic or go to a workshop.

The point is to start small and work the activity or habit into your life, stick with it, and move on to the next item on your list.

As you continue on your journey, don't forget to fully celebrate yourself and your wins along the way. Consistent action and effort in the right direction is a big deal, so celebrate it. Focus not just on the big goal and the time that it takes to accomplish it, but the strides you have made day by day. Take it one step at a time, give yourself grace, and trust the process. Whatever you do, don't give up.

A Healthier You Starts on the Inside

Food is an important component to improve our health. You want to make sure that you are eating properly and getting the required amounts of vitamins and minerals, ideally through food. There are times when supplements are necessary to ensure proper body function and health.

There are many vitamins and minerals that keep your body healthy. (See Chapter Six, Vitamins, Minerals, and Copper.) The next chapter will provide a quick overview of copper before we delve into its origins.

CHAPTER TWO

An Overview of Copper

At the mention of copper, the penny typically comes to mind. This unassuming coin may bring up a plethora of memories. From randomly finding a penny on the ground to purchasing candy or a toy for mere pennies, to making a wish before throwing one in a fountain, this coin evokes a different memory depending on the person and situation. Prior to 1982, pennies were made of approximately 95 percent copper. Thereafter, it was made with smaller traces of copper and mixed with zinc. The penny will always have a rare and distinctive look.

Copper will continue to impact our daily lives in many ways. This reddish-brown mineral is in nature, electrical and transportation equipment, plumbing material, wires, art, jewelry, and more. From its presence in our homes to its prevalence within earth's natural resources, copper has made its mark. As you can see, copper is necessary for many things to function properly. Copper also plays an important role in the human body, known to have many health and healing properties. Copper is an important element that is threaded through our everyday lives. It came from ancient times and will stand the test of time.

In the chapters of this book, you will learn about the origins of copper, how to incorporate copper into your diet, how the mineral can help heal the body, and more. The best way to consume copper is through food and/or supplements. There are many delicious foods with sufficient copper to give most people the daily recommended value of 900 micrograms (mcg) per day for the average adult.[2]

Consuming Copper

Small amounts of copper are naturally stored in the body. If you eat a well-balanced and nutrient-rich diet that includes foods with copper, it is easy to get the daily recommended amount of copper through food. The average amount that is naturally consumed through food is approximately 1,100 mcg for women and 1,300 mcg for men. This is a healthy amount and won't cause copper toxicity.

Due to the consumption of a lot of processed foods that lack nutrients, for some, it can be hard to get the proper amount of copper through foods. There are times when a copper deficiency can happen. A supplement can help ensure that copper is absorbed properly. Before taking any supplements, contact your doctor, and they can help you determine how much to take based on your age and the condition of your health, etc.

As mentioned, the daily recommendation for adults is 900 mcg of copper for both men and women.

Copper deficiencies are not common, but they can happen. If the body doesn't have enough copper, this can cause cardio-

---

2 "Office of Dietary Supplements—Copper," National Institutes of Health, last updated October 18, 2022, https://ods.od.nih.gov/factsheets/Copper -HealthProfessional.

vascular issues, such as weakness of the blood vessels and an irregular heartbeat, anemia, thyroid issues, osteoporosis, high cholesterol, bone fractures, a low white blood cell count, and the loss of skin pigmentation. Other symptoms include issues with brain development, weakened muscles, cold sensitivity, bone fractures, feeling fatigued or weak, frequent illness, premature gray hair, issues with memory, and vision loss.

Some health conditions can naturally cause copper levels to decrease and may result in a deficiency. Menkes disease and celiac disease are two such conditions. Like most minerals that are beneficial for your overall health and healing, copper needs to be consumed and absorbed properly. Some vitamins and minerals such as zinc, iron, and vitamin C are known to block the absorption of copper in the body if they are taken in high amounts.

The best way to get the proper amount of copper is through food, including the following:

o Almonds

o Avocado

o Beef liver

o Cashews

o Chia seeds

o Dark chocolate

o Goat cheese

o Kale

o Oysters

o Potatoes

o Quinoa

o Salmon

o Sesame seeds

o Spinach

o Sunflower seeds

o Turnip greens

It is rare to have copper toxicity, or too much copper in the body, but it can happen. Copper toxicity can result from taking vitamins that may contain more copper than the body needs. In addition, if some people have heavy levels of copper in their water, copper toxicity can occur. Some of the symptoms of copper toxicity include stomach pain, nausea, headache, heart complications, jaundice, and abnormalities with the red blood cells.

There are other minerals that work with copper to provide the greatest health benefit (see Chapter Eight, Copper Supplements). Consider this book your guide to all the wonderful ways copper can optimize your health and well-being.

But first, let's continue with an investigation into the origins of this essential mineral.

CHAPTER THREE

The Origins of Copper

Dating back over 10,000 years, copper is the first metal to be used by humans, giving the mineral a rich and compelling history. Users quickly learned that it was malleable and could be molded into different items such as tools, weapons, ornaments, and artisan crafts. Thus, copper was the metal that moved humans out of the Stone Age.

When copper was found and used, humans experimented with copper to find its proper and effective use. This is where they started to create tools, ornaments, weapons, and the like. As civilization continued, so did the utilization and growth of copper and other metals.

Copper holds great cultural significance in many areas of the world. For example, in Egypt, copper represents eternal life and was used in the Egyptian hieroglyphic system. In ancient times, the Egyptians were known to mine copper and make agricultural tools, housewares, and personal items. Some of the items that the Egyptians created were sickles, hoes, dishes, knives, razors, and mirrors. The Egyptians were also known to perfect the smelting and "lost-wax" method, where wax is used as a mold to shape an item. It is then covered in clay and the wax mold is melted and filled with molten copper.

The Romans used copper for coins, plumbing systems, and doors. The Romans also developed pipe organs made with copper. Copper is also widely used in the Middle East and Africa, where there have been early findings of the mineral dating back to approximately 900 BC. China, to date, is one of the world's largest importers of copper. In the past, the Chinese used copper and bronze for coins and other items. Copper also has a strong presence in Europe.

Copper was also used throughout history for health and healing.

For example, the Sumerians used copper for general medical purposes; the Chinese used copper topically for eye and skin diseases. They also gave copper orally for viruses and infections that affected the whole body. The ancient Indian culture used copper sulfate for general medical treatments; the Babylonian-Assyrians used copper bracelets and compounds containing copper for therapeutic healing. The Greeks were known to use copper to treat eye diseases as well as vaginal, gastrointestinal, and pulmonary disorders. They also used copper bracelets for arthritis. The Mayan, Aztec, and Incan cultures used copper sulfate-soaked gauzes to help reduce the bacteria and disinfect surgical wounds. The ancient Roman culture used numerous copper compounds topically to help treat wounds, inflamed tonsils, hemorrhoids, as well as skin and eye diseases. Throughout Africa copper was used for medicinal purposes such as healing treatments for illnesses, skin diseases, and sores. This is a brief overview of some of the specific ways that copper was used in different countries and cultures.

Copper is found in different parts of the world. Some of the areas include Peru, Chile, Canada, Russia, and Africa. The United States is noted as the second largest producer of copper. Some of the major mines in the states are found in Michigan, Montana, Arizona, and New Mexico.

Today, as you can see, copper continues to impact our daily lives throughout many industries. One of the many ways copper is still used today is for its health and healing properties.

Before we get into those benefits for the body, it is important to understand what copper is and where it came from. This short chapter explains the origins of copper and some of its uses in various industries.

The Basics of Copper

The term "copper" comes from the Latin term *cuprum*. Copper is a chemical element with a reddish-brown hue. With the symbol of Cu and sitting at number 29 on the periodic table, this unassuming metal has its place in our environment, electrical units, industrial industries, currency, and more.

Copper Alloys

Due to its texture, copper is often used as an alloy, a material that consists of two combined metals or of a metal and a nonmetal material. Alloys are known to make singular metals stronger.

For example, two common copper alloys are brass and bronze. Brass is a mixture of copper and zinc, and bronze is a mixture of copper and tin. Other alloys include manganese, gold, nickel, and phosphorus, just to name a few. The penny is primarily made from zinc and covered with copper.

To determine if copper is real: in general copper is known to repel magnets. In addition, copper has a hue that is reddish in nature and to some may have hints of an orangish or pink hue. Since copper is a soft metal, the sound of copper is typically muted. If you hear a ringing bell-type sound, it is probably an alloy.

When metals are combined, they can make a number of different items, such as musical instruments, heat exchangers or systems that transfer heat, pipelines, screw propellers, which are rotating blades that help to push air and water, and more.

Around 4000 BC, the Egyptians used two copper compounds, malachite and azurite, to make items resulting in a green and blue makeup. Copper in Egypt was often mixed with iron or zinc. In order to make tin, the Egyptians also mixed copper with bronze. The Egyptians found ways to mix copper with other metals so the texture could stay strong for tools and goods such as statues, dishes, trays, weapons, ornaments, and more.

The Romans used an alloy of copper and zinc, which has become what we know as brass. The material was used to create coins, parts of doors, pipe organs, and sections of plumbing pipes.

Today copper is still used in many ways, from essential items to specialty items, and from cultural traditions to healing.

Copper and the Home

Copper is present in art, jewelry, musical instruments, coins, home décor items, kitchen utensils, vacuum tubes, plumbing, sinks, and more.

Copper and the Environment

Copper is one of the most effectively recycled metals. About one-third of all of the copper used worldwide is recycled. Due to the strength of the metal, it will not lose any of its physical or chemical properties when it is repurposed or mixed with alloys.

Copper and Electrical Units

Copper is popular with electrical wiring due to its corrosion resistance. Some familiar electrical systems that we use copper in include telecommunications wiring, modems, and routers.

Copper and Transportation

The auto, aviation, and train industries are heavily reliant on copper due to its thermal and electric properties. You can also find copper in items such as brakes, radiators, connectors, wiring, and motors. A car has approximately 50 pounds of copper. [3]

Copper and Metaphysics

Copper is known for its health and healing properties in the body. Copper is also used in the metaphysical world. Copper offers benefits such as balancing and serving as a guard against negative energies. Copper is also known to align your energetic field and body for strength and stamina and to balance your chakras. Simply wearing copper, holding it during meditation, and/or using it during energetic treatments such as Reiki is known to benefit healing and energy from a metaphysical standpoint.

---

3 "Copper Facts: Copper in Transportation," Copper Facts: Copper in Transportation, accessed October 20, 2022, https://www.copper.org /education/c-facts/transportation/print-category.html.

Copper and Construction

Copper has also been in construction for a long time, from doors to doorknobs, handles, gates, bathroom fixtures, faucets, and more.

Copper in the Health Industry

Copper is also needed for the body to properly function. We will discuss this in more detail in the chapters to come.

This is a very brief overview of copper and some of its significance throughout the world. There is so much more to learn about the history and cultural significance of this metal. The focus of this book is on the health and healing benefits of copper. Let's dive in!

CHAPTER FOUR

The Healing Properties of Copper

Copper offers many health benefits to the body. It is easy to get the daily recommended amount of 900 micrograms (mcg) per day for the average adult and 1,300 mcg a day for women who are pregnant or lactating. Babies and children from birth to twelve months should consume 200 mcg of copper per day; children one to three years old, 340 mcg; children four to eight years old, 440 mcg; children nine to thirteen years old, 700 mcg; and children fourteen to eighteen years old, 890 mcg.[4]

Most people can consume these amounts through food alone if they consume a nutrient-rich diet with a good mixture of fruits and vegetables. If you eat a diet with a lot of processed foods with high levels of sodium and sugar, it will be difficult to consume the daily amount of copper because many of these foods don't have a lot of nutritional value. If you eat a healthy balanced diet and include foods that have copper, you will most likely consume enough copper to help your body function prop-

---

4 "Office of Dietary Supplements—Copper," last updated October 18, 2022.

erly. If you don't meet the daily requirements and your copper levels are low, supplements are available.

Although the recommended levels are easy to attain, a copper deficiency can occur. A copper deficiency can be caused by not consuming the right amounts of the mineral through foods. Another reason is taking zinc supplements because it competes with copper to absorb properly in the body. Stomach surgery can also cause a copper deficiency. In addition, some health conditions like Menkes disease and celiac disease can also cause a copper deficiency.

Too much copper in the body can lead to toxicity, inflammation, and certain health conditions. Copper toxicity can happen through consuming contaminated water that has high levels of copper and an overconsumption of copper supplementation. It is important to check with your doctor regarding your levels of copper. You can find out your levels through a blood test and a ceruloplasmin test. This is a test that measures the levels of ceruloplasmin, a protein that aids in distributing copper in the bloodstream. These tests are helpful, so you won't have issues with copper deficiency or copper toxicity.

The Health Benefits of Copper

When adequate amounts of copper are present in the body, the highest levels of copper are typically found in the brain and liver. Other areas where copper is found include the heart, pancreas, and kidneys. During pregnancy, copper levels are typically higher because estrogen is known to increase the amounts of copper in the body.

Overall, copper is known to help to form hemoglobin, it aids in the absorption of iron from the intestines, and it is needed to produce energy in the body. Copper also helps the body in several ways. This includes:

o Helping the production of red blood cells

o Absorbing iron in the body

o Forming collagen

o Regulating blood pressure and heart rate

o Reducing inflammation

o Helping to maintain the strength of the organs and the connective tissue

o Helps energy levels

o Helps brain function

o Enhances the formation of collagen and the overall health of skin and hair

o Developing, maintaining, and sustaining connective tissue and the bones

o Improves health conditions related to the immune system

There are some enzymes that are also dependent on copper to function. One in particular is tyrosinase, which is used in the formation of melanin, which is responsible for your eye, hair, and skin pigmentation. Copper is also known to help other health conditions such as arthritis, heart conditions, thyroid health, and neurological health.[5]

---

5 "Copper," Linus Pauling Institute, accessed August 3, 2022, https://lpi .oregonstate.edu/mic/minerals/copper.

Next, we'll discuss in more detail the specific ways that copper can help the health and healing of the body.

Joint and Bone Health

Bone health keeps our bodies moving properly. When the bones are healthy it can also help the immune system. In addition, as aging progresses, bone health is very important. Aging can cause low bone density, which weakens the bones. This can cause an increased risk of fractures. There are other bone-related conditions that can cause stress on the body, such as different forms of arthritis.

Some ways to maintain bone health include exercise, proper stretching, and consuming the proper nutrients that help bone health. In addition to copper, this includes vitamin D, potassium, protein, vitamin C, zinc, and calcium. Collectively, these vitamins and minerals can be consumed through foods such as prunes, avocados, tomatoes, cheese, and milk. Some foods such as fried foods, highly processed foods, alcohol, and sugar can speed up the bone deterioration process and increase inflammation. This can lead to osteoporosis and other forms of arthritis.

The body depends on copper for the healthy formation of connective tissue. In addition, copper is the mineral that is responsible for linking elastin and collagen, which help the mobility of the body and aid in the prevention of brakes and fractures.

Another way that copper helps the bones is by interacting with iron, zinc, and manganese to create an antioxidant called superoxide dismutase. This antioxidant protects and saves bones from damage caused by oxidative stress. It also helps the bones in the body sustain their strength and movement while preventing easy breakage. If copper is not combined with iron, manganese, and zinc, the antioxidant superoxide dismutase can't form in the body properly and the bone protection that it should provide is not as effective. Bone health is important for our skeletal system and strong bones can help prevent bone and muscular-related conditions.[6]

Long-term copper deficiency can cause weak and brittle bones. As the bones weaken over a long period of time and the cartilage wears, different forms of arthritis may arise. One common form of arthritis that occurs due to poor bone health is osteoporosis. This condition primarily affects the spine, hips, or wrist. When a person has osteoporosis, new bone development doesn't keep up to replace the old bones of the affected area, leaving them weak and brittle. Proper copper levels in the body are known to aid in the reduction of osteoporosis. Other factors may affect the health of bones negatively. This includes taking medication that can cause bone damage and having other health conditions that affect the bones.

In general, when copper levels are low, bone strength is weakened. Along with calcium, copper can help keep bones strong and functioning well. Research suggests that a diet that is high in refined flour, fructose, and sugar has the potential to interfere with copper absorption.[7]

---

6 Charles T. Price, Joshua R. Langford, and Frank A. Liporace, "Essential Nutrients for Bone Health and a Review of Their Availability in the Average North American Diet," *The Open Orthopaedics Journal* 6, no. 1 (2012): 143–149, doi:10.2174/1874325001206010143.

7 Nathaniel H. O. Harder et al., "Effects of Dietary Glucose and Fructose on Copper, Iron, and Zinc Metabolism Parameters in Humans," *Nutrients* 12 no. 9 (2020): 2581, doi:10.3390/nu12092581.

Collagen and Connective Tissue

Copper helps the connective tissue, which binds, supports, and connects specific tissues in the body. There are three categories of connective tissue:

o Dense connective tissue: consists of ligaments and tendons with a larger density of collagen

o Specialized connective tissue: consists of bone, blood, and lymph.

o Loose connective tissue: assists with holding the organs in place. It is made up of reticular fibers, extracellular matrix, and collagen.

Copper also aids the formation of collagen by activating and linking to lysyl oxidase, an enzyme that is needed to aid in the strengthening and formation of collagen. It also has a role in the production and protection of the connective tissue by crosslinking the collagen, elastin, and extracellular matrix proteins. This also plays a part in keeping the heart and blood vessels healthy. If there is a copper deficiency, lysyl oxidase can't properly function in the body.[8]

Along with proper nutrition that includes vitamins and minerals that support bone and joint health, regular exercise, stretching, and eating a healthy diet can also help the bones and joints.[9]

---

8 "Ciba Foundation Symposium 79—Biological Roles of Copper," *Novartis Foundation Symposia*, (1980), doi:10.1002/9780470720622.

9 Payvand Kamrani, Geoffrey Marston, and Arif Jan, "Anatomy, Connective Tissue," National Institutes of Health, January 24, 2022, https://www.ncbi.nlm.nih.gov/books/NBK538534.

Hair, Skin, and Nails

Copper is a mineral that is known to enhance the hair, skin, and nails with the help of copper peptides. Copper peptides are small chains of amino acids that build protein and aid in producing elastin and collagen. Copper peptides work below the epidermis, or outer layer of the skin and aid in the production of elastin deep within the skin tissues.

The skin has three layers of tissues: the epidermis, the dermis, and the subcutaneous layer. The epidermis is the outer layer of the skin that also has the cells that contain melanin, or melanocytes. The top portion or outer layer of the epidermis is a very thin layer and consists of the dead cells that wash off. The dead cells are replaced by new cells that are produced in the lower portion of the epidermis.

The middle layer of the skin is the dermis. This layer contains hair follicles, sweat glands, oil glands, blood vessels, and nerves. The dermis is also made up of elastic fibers and collagen, the agents that give the skin elasticity and strength.

The deepest layer of the skin is the subcutaneous layer. This has blood vessels, nerves, and fatty tissue. The fatty tissue from this layer protects the body from extreme heat and cold and helps protect the body from injuries.

Copper is also known for its anti-aging effects. It protects the skin against free radicals and inflammation. It also reduces the appearance of wrinkles and evens out the skin tone while reducing age spots, uneven skin, and acne scars.

Copper benefits the hair because it is a mineral that is needed to produce melanin, a compound that is responsible for the color of your eyes, skin, and hair. Research has also shown that copper helps to maintain tissues in the blood vessels and increase the blood circulation in the skin and scalp. (See Hair and Skin on page 59.)

Along with the skin and hair, copper aids in keeping the nails strong and healthy. This is due to the supportive growth of the keratinocytes, which is the main cell of the epidermis.[10]

Beautiful hair, skin, and nails start from the inside out. Drinking water, eating a healthy diet, exercising, and getting the proper amount of rest will naturally help the appearance of your hair, skin, and nails. Using additional personal care items such as cosmetics, lotions, serums, and moisturizers will enhance your natural beauty.[11]

Thyroid Gland

The thyroid gland is responsible for the production and regulation of hormones. The thyroid gland helps brain development, bone maintenance, digestive function, heart muscle function, and the body's metabolic rate. Copper is an important mineral for thyroid metabolism, particularly when it comes to hormone absorption and production.

Copper is known to activate the production of thyroxine hormone, also known as T4, while helping the body by prevent-

10 Loren Pickart and Anna Margolina, "Regenerative and Protective Actions of the GHK-Cu Peptide in the Light of the New Gene Data," *International Journal of Molecular Sciences* 19, no. 7 (2018): 1987, doi:10.3390/ijms1907 1987.

11 Gadi Borkow, "Using Copper to Improve the Well-Being of the Skin," *Current Chemical Biology* 8, no. 2 (2015): 89–102, doi:10.2174/2212796809 666150227223857.

ing it from overabsorbing this hormone in the blood cells. This is done by copper helping the body control calcium levels.

Copper also helps the synthesis of phospholipids. These are molecules that are a major component of cell membranes that are known to reinvigorate the thyroid-stimulating hormone. Phospholipids are also known to aid in supporting mitochondrial function, liver health, and the strength of the gut lining.[12]

Healing Treatment for Cancer

There are reports that show that high levels of copper can cause cancer and that copper also has some healing agents that can aid in reducing cancerous tumors.

Although this topic is still being researched, there are reports that show that high levels of copper in the blood are linked to several types of cancer, including lung, cervix, brain, liver, and breast cancer.[13] In addition, research shows that some cancer cells have higher levels of copper, and copper may play role in developing tumors.

Although high levels of copper may be linked to cancer, studies have also found that copper can have antitumor effects. One way to remove metals out of the body is through chelation therapy. This is a process of administering medicine through the bloodstream. The medicine bonds the metals, the metals filters

12 Manisha Arora, "Study of Trace Elements in Patients of Hypothyroidism With Special Reference to Zinc and Copper," *Biomedical Journal of Scientific & Technical Research* 6, no. 2 (2018), doi:10.26717/bjstr.2018.06.001336.

13 A. Hordyjewska, Ł. Popiołek, and J. Kocot, "The Many 'Faces' of Copper in Medicine and Treatment," *Biometals: An International Journal on the Role of Metal Ions in Biology, Biochemistry, and Medicine* 27, no. 4 (2014): 611–621, https://doi.org/10.1007/s10534-014-9736-5.

into kidneys, and it is released through the urine. Another way copper is known to aid in reducing tumors is with copper salts—this helps by aiding in breaking down damaged proteins and inducing antitumor effects.[14]

Energy and the Immune System

It is important to have enough energy to carry out your daily tasks. There is nothing like an extra dose of energy throughout the day. There are a number of ways to keep your energy levels balanced. Generally, eating healthy, exercising, getting proper sleep, and engaging in activities that you enjoy are all known to increase energy. Copper can also help your energy levels.

Copper helps to metabolize iron in the body. This helps energy production while keeping the blood vessels healthy. Copper is also a cofactor, a chemical that is not a protein that aids with biological chemical reactions, of many enzymes that help produce energy throughout the body.

Copper also helps the development and maintenance of the immune system. It interacts with other cells to keep the immune system healthy. A copper deficiency may cause a deficiency of neutrophils, white blood cells that fight off infection. This can lead to a lot of health conditions and make it difficult to heal when you are sick or injured.[15]

---

14 Francesco Tisato et al., "Copper in Diseases and Treatments, and Copper-Based Anticancer Strategies," *Medicinal Research Reviews* 10, no. 4 (2010): 708–749, doi:10.1002/med.20174.

15 Karrera Y. Djoko et al., "The Role of Copper and Zinc Toxicity in Innate Immune Defense Against Bacterial Pathogens," *Journal of Biological Chemistry* 290, no. 31 (2015): 18954–18961, doi:10.1074/jbc.r115.647099.

Weight Loss

There is no quick fix for long-term weight loss. It requires a lifestyle change and making the choice to sustain these changes. There are some vitamins and minerals that can help you maintain and sustain health. Getting the proper nutrients that you need in the body can help you stop craving unhealthy snacks and foods.

Copper may have a boosting effect when it comes to weight loss. Studies have shown that copper may have the ability to break down an enzyme called PDE3. This enzyme is known to reduce the body's fat-burning ability. Research has shown that copper can block the enzyme cyclic adenosine monophosphate (cAMP) from binding to PDE3 and this allows the body to naturally break down fat. Although this finding is hopeful, the studies on this are not fully conclusive, so more research has to be conducted.

Brain Health

Copper is essential for proper brain function because the demand for oxygen is strongly dependent on copper. When it comes to copper and brain health, balance is important. Although the brain has a natural function that regulates copper metabolism, too much or too little copper can impact the brain negatively. Brain health requires more than vitamins and minerals. Other ways to keep your brain healthy include engaging in intellectually stimulating activities, exercising, getting enough sleep, listening to music, and maintaining a healthy social life.

Heart Health

The main function of the heart is to transport blood and nutrients throughout the body. A healthy heart is essential for a healthy circulatory system. Overall, keeping active with a regular exercise schedule, maintaining a healthy diet, getting adequate sleep, and finding ways to decrease stress are all wonderful ways to keep the heart healthy. Copper is a mineral that can improve heart health.

Studies have shown that copper can reduce stress on the heart by preventing many heart-related diseases and promoting heart strength. Copper has the ability to prevent the enlargement of an overworked heart due to stress. Studies have also shown that individuals who have copper deficiencies are known to be more susceptible to clot formation, heart disease, oxidative tissue damage, and increased cholesterol. This same study shows that the cardiac tissue biopsies of heart attack victims have a large reduction of copper levels in the body.[16]

People who have low copper levels in the body are known to have higher blood pressure levels, high cholesterol, and increased uric acid levels. Collectively this can lead to many health conditions such as heart disease, stroke, gout, kidney stones, and issues with proper kidney function.

Getting proper amounts of copper through food and supplements, if needed, can help maintain proper copper levels. Although low copper levels can play a part in the above health conditions, there are many other factors that can lead to them. It is important to check with your doctor to examine your medical

---

16 Hema Bashyam, "Heavy Metal for a Troubled Heart," *Journal of Experimental Medicine* 204, no. 3 (2007): 455a, doi:10.1084/jem.2043iti5.

history, physical health, levels of vitamins and minerals in the body, and symptoms of related illnesses.

To keep the heart functioning properly, it is important to exercise, reduce stress, eat a healthy diet, and refrain from overindulging in salt, sugar, and processed foods. It is also important to minimize alcohol intake and refrain from smoking.

Copper Toxicity

You can have too much copper in the body. There are a number of ways that copper toxicity can happen. One way is consuming water that has high levels of copper. High levels of copper in the water can come from pipes and copper alloys in plumbing. Public water systems do have an upper limit for copper that is established by the Environmental Protection Agency. When people consume water with high levels of copper this typically comes from the faucet or pipes in the home. As the faucets and pipes age and break down, the metal can seep into the water.

Some people may consume too much copper by taking too many supplements, not realizing how much copper is in them. Some supplements just have copper and others have copper mixed in with other vitamins and minerals.

Although copper toxicity is rare, there are symptoms that indicate that there is too much copper in the body. Symptoms of chronic exposure to high levels of copper include abdominal pain, nausea, vomiting, diarrhea, and cramps. More severe symptoms include kidney failure, heart failure, brain disorders, and liver damage.

Wilson's disease is also linked to copper toxicity. Wilson's disease is a rare and genetic medical condition that causes copper to accumulate in the organs and prevents the body from getting rid of the accumulated copper. These organs include the brain, liver, corneas of the eye, and other vital organs. Symptoms of Wilson's disease include issues with walking and coordination, pain in the abdomen, swollen blood vessels, swelling, tremors, and extreme fatigue.

Treatment of copper toxicity consists of four major focus areas: observation of the patient, specific management of the complications conducted by a healthcare professional, the reduction of absorption of copper, and chelation therapy, a medical procedure that aids in removing heavy metals from the body. When a person gets chelation therapy, this treatment can be given through an intravenous tube (IV) or via pill form. When a person gets chelation therapy, the drug binds metals in the blood. Once the medication is attached to the metal, the body will remove the metals through urination.[17]

Copper Deficiency

As stated before, copper deficiency, or hypocupremia, is rare, but it does happen. It is also often misdiagnosed. This is because some of the symptoms of a copper deficiency present similar to a deficiency of vitamins and minerals that require higher levels in the body.

For example, a copper deficiency may present similar to a vitamin B-12 deficiency, folate deficiency, anemia, and neutro-

---

17 "Office of Dietary Supplements—Copper," last updated October 18, 2022.

penia, which is a reduction in neuropils, a white blood cell that is needed to help fight infection. To find out if you have a copper deficiency, your doctor can administer a blood test for plasma copper levels. If a person has less than 30 percent of the recommended copper levels, then they are considered severely deficient.[18]

One of the most common causes of a copper deficiency is malabsorption. Gastric bypass surgery is known to be one of the most common causes of acquired copper malabsorption. This is because when people get this surgery it leads to insufficient gastrointestinal absorption, which is also a common cause of copper deficiency. Another cause of copper deficiency is high levels of zinc in the body. Whether it is through diet or taking a supplement, zinc and copper are both absorbed in the proximal duodenum, the first part of the small intestine and the stomach.

When there are large amounts of zinc in the stomach, the excess causes an increased production of metallothionein. Copper binds to the metallothionein and excretes through the intestinal tract.[19]

Another mineral that can potentially cause a copper deficiency at high levels is iron. Researchers found that high levels of iron in rats caused a copper deficiency. In the finding, they reported that high levels of iron interrupted the natural ability of the body to distribute copper in the tissues and control copper absorption

18 Shoaib M. Wazir and Ibrahim Ghobrial, "Copper Deficiency, A New Triad: Anemia, Leucopenia, and Myeloneuropathy," *Journal of Community Hospital Internal Medicine Perspectives* 7, no. 4 (2017): 265–268, doi:10.1080/200096 66.2017.1351289.

19 Harry N. Hoffman, Robert L. Phyliky and C. Richard Fleming, "Zinc-Induced Copper Deficiency," *Gastroenterology* 94, no. 2 (1988): 508–512, doi:10.1016/0016-5085(88)90445-3.

in the intestines. There are continuous studies being conducted to get a full determination of whether or not high levels of iron, in fact, is a cause of a copper deficiency.

The following health conditions can also cause a reduction of copper levels in the body and lead to a deficiency.

Celiac Disease

Celiac disease is a digestive and immune disorder that may affect several organs in the body, mainly the small intestine. With this disorder, gluten can cause issues in the digestive system. The body doesn't get the proper nutrients that it needs. Since copper is primarily absorbed in the small intestine, this can create a deficiency of the mineral.[20]

Crohn's Disease

Crohn's disease is a condition that causes inflammation of the digestive tract. Crohn's is a type of inflammatory bowel disease that can cause extreme fatigue, weight loss, malnutrition, and abdominal pain. Studies show that individuals with Crohn's are known to have insufficient amounts of zinc and copper.[21]

Irritable Bowel Syndrome (IBS)

Irritable bowel syndrome is a gastrointestinal disorder that causes pain in the abdomen, constipation, gas, diarrhea, and

---

20 Brent P. Goodman et al., "Copper Deficiency Myeloneuropathy Due to Occult Celiac Disease," *The Neurologist* 15, no. 6 (2009): 355c356, doi:10.1097/nrl.0b013e31819428a8.

21 Tobias Schneider et al., "The Copper/Zinc Ratio Correlates with Markers of Disease Activity in Patients with Inflammatory Bowel Disease," *Crohn's & Colitis* 2, no. 1 (2020), https://doi.org/10.1093/crocol/otaa001.

changes in the bowel movements. Some of the causes of this condition include visceral hypersensitivity or extra-sensitive nerves in the gastrointestinal (GI) tract. This causes issues with the way that food moves through the GI tract and can also create a miscommunication between the brain, gut, and nerves. Studies have shown that there is a copper imbalance in individuals who have irritable bowel syndrome.[22]

Menkes Disease

Menkes disease is a genetic disorder that causes a defect in the ATP7A gene. There are times when Menkes disease is not inherited and the condition occurs when the baby is conceived. Studies have shown that Menkes disease affects one out of every 100,000 to 250,000 live births worldwide. Symptoms include low body temperature, seizures, delayed weight gain and growth, jaundice, and saggy facial features.

When a person has this condition, it affects the body's ability to make a protein that enables copper to properly distribute throughout the body. Instead, copper builds up in the kidneys and small intestines. Although there is no cure, treatments with copper can help reduce the symptoms of Menkes disease.[23]

---

22 Isabel A. Hujoel and Margaux L. A. Hujoel, "The Role of Copper and Zinc in Irritable Bowel Syndrome: A Mendelian Randomization Study," *American Journal of Epidemiology* 191, no. 1 (2021): 85–92, doi:10.1093/aje/kwab180.

23 "Menkes Disease—NORD (National Organization for Rare Disorders)," NORD (National Organization for Rare Disorders), 2020, https://rarediseases.org/rare-diseases/menkes-disease.

Symptoms of Low Copper Levels

Low copper levels can affect the immune system, energy levels, and overall health. Some of the symptoms of low copper levels in the body include the following:

o Abnormal lipid levels

o Anemia

o Arthritis

o Ataxia (Poor muscle control that causes uncontrolled movements. It can cause difficulty with balance and walking, speech, eye movements, and hand coordination.)

o Higher blood cholesterol levels

o Connective tissue disorders

o Consistently feeling cold

o Easy bone breakage

o Easy bruising

o Fatigue

o Getting sick easily or frequently

o Hypopigmentation

o Inflammation in the body

o Pancytopenia (A condition where a person has a highly reduced number of white blood cells, red blood cells, and platelets.)

o Skin sores

o Unexplained muscle soreness

Treatment

To treat a copper deficiency, your doctor will most likely suggest a copper supplement. If the deficiency is severe, an IV may be required. It typically takes 4 to 12 weeks to get the copper levels at a healthy level in the body.

It is important to have a conversation with your doctor regarding your vitamin and mineral levels. If you find that your levels are too low or too high, your doctor can help you with a plan that works for you.

CHAPTER FIVE

Wearing Copper

In addition to consuming copper through foods and supplements for its health and healing benefits, wearing copper is known to aid in healing areas of the body, improve the skin, and provide relief from ailments such as sore muscles and arthritis. Some of the copper-containing items that people wear include jewelry, clothing, cosmetics, and skin products.

Jewelry and Copper

Who doesn't love a statement piece of jewelry? It is a great conversation starter and depending on the specific item, a beautiful piece of artwork. For some, it is a special heirloom that is passed down from generation to generation. Some people see jewelry as an accessory for an outfit. For others, it has a deeper meaning, and some people keep jewelry as a collector's item. Jewelry can also be used as a healing tool.

Wearing copper bracelets for healing practices started around the eighth century BC. Throughout the years, copper jewelry is commonly used to treat pain, particularly bracelets and rings.

When individuals wear copper jewelry, it undergoes an oxidation process during which small amounts of the mineral absorb into the skin and enter the bloodstream. The skin is the largest organ on the body and absorbs many of the items that we apply topically. Some people shy away from wearing copper because at times it can turn the skin green. This is because of oxidation—when a chemical is mixed with oxygen, oxidation occurs. So, when copper naturally reacts to the body's chemical balance due to the oil, sweat, and natural acidic composition of the body, the copper jewelry that is worn can turn the skin green. Depending on the wearer's skin tone, the color of the copper stain will vary in color. This stain can easily be removed with soap and water.

In holistic health and spiritual practices, the copper coloration on the skin can help to determine a person's levels of stress, acidity, and the ways that diet is impacting the body.

Although many people wear copper jewelry for its healing properties, one study followed sixty-five participants with rheumatoid arthritis who wore a copper bracelet or magnetic wrist strap for five weeks. In their self-reported results, the study concluded that there wasn't a big difference in reducing arthritis symptoms. If there was any change in the arthritis condition of the participants due to wearing the jewelry, researchers found it was primarily with the placebo effect of participants who had rheumatoid arthritis.[24]

---

24 Stewart J. Richmond et al., "Copper Bracelets and Magnetic Wrist Straps for Rheumatoid Arthritis—Analgesic and Anti-Inflammatory Effects: A Randomised Double-Blind Placebo Controlled Crossover Trial," *Plos ONE* 8, no. 9 (2013): e71529, doi:10.1371/journal.pone.0071529.

Cleaning Copper Jewelry

If you have copper jewelry for healing purposes or in general, there are a few ways that you can keep it clean. The easiest way is with warm, soapy water. The other ways are easy and you can find the ingredients right in the kitchen.

o **Baking soda** is a great product to clean copper with. Combine four tablespoons of baking soda with one tablespoon of water. A paste will form. Apply this paste on your copper jewelry and let it sit for about five minutes. Scrub the jewelry with a microfiber cloth or toothbrush.

o **Ketchup** is not just for adding flavor to your food. Ketchup does wonders for cleaning copper. Put the ketchup all over the copper jewelry. Once it dries, use a clean cloth to clean the jewelry, wash it with soap, and dry it.

o **Lemons** are a good option for cleaning copper. Take a lemon, cut it in half, put salt on the lemon, and rub your jewelry with it. Another way is to squeeze the lemon juice and add salt to a bowl. The ratio should be 75 percent lemon and 25 percent salt. To avoid scratches from the salt, make sure that the salt is fully dissolved in the lemon juice. Take a clean toothbrush or cloth, put it in the solution, and rub your jewelry with the toothbrush or cloth.

o **Vinegar** is a great choice for cleaning a lot of items such as glass, windows, floors, walls, sinks, and, of course, copper. To clean your copperware and/or jewelry, simply put two tablespoons of salt with a cup of vinegar. Put your copper jewelry in the solution and let it soak for thirty minutes. Once the soaking is complete, you can pat it dry and let it air dry or gently scrub it with a toothbrush, soap, and water.

Copper Clothing

Copper-infused clothing and other items such as braces for the knees, elbows, ankles, and hands, socks, wound dressings, and bedding have also gained much popularity over the years. Items that include copper have copper oxide particles that are infused into the textile products and are used as a holding space for copper ions. When there is a presence of humidity or moisture, the copper ions are spread through the product

Some of the findings of using some of these wearable items that have copper include improvements in the appearance of skin and some ailments. For example, in a study of fifty-six participants who had acute or chronic athlete's foot infections, the participants wore socks containing copper for eight hours a day. The results showed that within eight to twelve days the symptoms of athlete's foot showed improvement or resolution. Symptoms that improved include burning, eruptions, scaling, itching, and/or erythema or redness of the skin. In this study, there were 21 diabetic patients. The type of diabetes among the patients was not specified. Diabetes reduces the ability to improve infections and skin damage. The study showed that the skin looked healthier in areas of the foot where there was no fungal infection.

In a clinical trial that was conducted, a group of participants ages 30 to 60 used a copper oxide pillowcase while another group used pillowcases that didn't contain copper oxide. According to the study the test participants used the pillowcase for 4 and 8 weeks. Both groups also used face cleansers and moisturizers. The studies found that the group that used the copper oxide pillowcases had a higher reduction of wrinkles and an improved

58

overall skin appearance after using the pillowcases during the four and eight weeks.[25]

Hair and Skin

Copper is known to enhance the appearance of both the skin and hair, making it a staple in the beauty industry from historic times to the present day.

Many facial serums, creams, moisturizers, lotions, makeup products, and a plethora of personal care products contain copper.[26] Some of the beauty benefits that copper offers include increasing the appearance of the skin by strengthening elasticity and smoothness, as well as offering skin protection. This is due to the copper peptides that work as an antioxidant by protecting the skin against free radicals and reducing inflammation.

The hair can also benefit from copper. This metal is known to help the hair grow, increase the thickness of the hair, increase the size of the hair follicles, and reduce the speed of growth of gray hair.

Many beauty products such as eye creams, face masks, moisturizers, serums, and some lip balms contain copper peptides, which are the small chains of amino acids that build protein. If you want to utilize the benefits of these products, some of the

---

25 Ji Hwoon Baek et al., "Reduction of Facial Wrinkles Depth by Sleeping on Copper Oxide-Containing Pillowcases: A Double Blind, Placebo Controlled, Parallel, Randomized Clinical Study," *Journal of Cosmetic Dermatology* 11, no. 3 (2012): 193–200, https://doi.org/10.1111/j.1473-2165.2012.00624.x.

26 Gadi Borkow, "Using Copper to Improve the Well-Being of the Skin," *Current Chemical Biology* 8, no. 2 (2015): 89–102, doi:10.2174/2212796809 666150227223857.

following ingredients that include copper peptides are the following:

- copper tripeptide
- copper amino
- copper lysine
- copper lysinate/prolinate
- GHK-Cu or copper gluconate

Some ingredients are known to reduce the full benefit of copper peptides on the skin. These ingredients are retinol, vitamin C, glycolic acid, and alpha hydroxy acids (AHAs). Although these are very popular components of skincare treatments and will benefit the skin, it is not advised to use them together with copper peptides. Use products with copper peptides separate from the others.[27]

Skin

The skin is the largest organ of the body. It is important to maintain the health of the skin. It is known as a defender against bacteria that could enter the body and affect internal organs. The skin also aids in keeping the immune system healthy and regulating the body's temperature.

Eating properly, taking skin-enhancing vitamins and minerals such as vitamins C, D, E, K, copper, selenium, and zinc, undertaking a regular exercise regime, reducing stress, and avoiding highly processed and sugary foods will help your skin and overall health.

---

27 "What Is GHK-Cu (Copper Peptide) and How Does It Work?" *Peptidesciences.com*, 2022, https://www.peptidesciences.com/blog/what-is -ghk-cu-and-how.

Some products on the market with copper peptides are beneficial for the skin. If you get the proper daily recommended amount of copper, 15 percent of copper is found in the skin. Copper benefits the skin in the following ways:

o Enhances the collagen

o Gives skin a clear and firm appearance

o Increases the elasticity of the skin

o Increases wound healing

o Improves the appearance of the skin

o Improves the structure of aging skin

o Protects skin and skin cells from UV radiation

o Reduces inflammation

o Reduces fine lines and wrinkles

o Reduces rough and dry skin

o Reduces the damage of free radicals

o Reduces skin spots, acne scars, and hyperpigmentation

o Reverses thinning skin

o Stabilizes skin proteins[28]

Along with topical skin products, copper-infused household items can potentially help the skin as well. There was a study that showed that copper-embedded pillowcases, wound dressings, and socks helped the skin's elasticity, aided in the cure of

28 Charles T. Price, Joshua R. Langford and Frank A. Liporace, "Essential Nutrients for Bone Health and a Review of Their Availability in the Average North American Diet," *The Open Orthopaedics Journal* 6, no. 1 (2012): 143–149, doi:10.2174/1874325001206010143.

athlete's foot infection, aided in wound healing, and reduced wrinkles and fine lines on the face.[29]

Though copper can benefit the skin, remember it is not a cure-all. Think of it as a great way to enhance and improve your overall skin health.

Hair

Hair from head to toe offers several benefits to the body. Just like the skin, it can offer protection. The hair on our heads and bodies can protect us from sweat, dust, dirt, and sun. Our hair also helps us with the regulation of body temperature.

Each hair has a root and a shaft. The root is surrounded by the hair follicle and the shaft is the part that sticks out of the skin. Copper peptides are known to stimulate the capillaries under the scalp, which in turn creates healthy blood circulation to the scalp and aids in healthy hair growth. They also promote hair thickness and hair strength, aiding in the prevention of hair loss, shedding, and follicle death. Copper peptides also block dihydrotestosterone (DHT), a hormone that is a cause of male hair loss.[30] In addition to promoting scalp health, according to some alternative healing theories, copper can reduce gray hair growth. Although this is not fully confirmed by research, it's theorized that melanin production spurred by copper is the cause.

Copper is a beneficial metal for health and beauty.

---

29 "Healthy Skin," American Skin Association, accessed November 8, 2022, https://www.americanskin.org/resource.

30 Hyun Keol Pyo et al., "The Effect of Tripeptide-Copper Complex on Human Hair Growth in Vitro," *Archives of Pharmacal Research* 30, no. 7 (2007): 834–839, doi:10.1007/bf02978833.

CHAPTER SIX

Vitamins, Minerals, and Copper

We commonly hear the advice to take our vitamins and minerals so we can stay healthy. Many people have their go-to supplement that they take daily or throughout the week. When we take vitamins and minerals, it is important to know the amount that we have in our bodies. It is also important to know which vitamins and minerals should be combined so they can properly be absorbed in the body. For example, vitamin C helps to absorb iron, and vitamin D helps absorb calcium.

If a doctor recommends supplements due to a copper deficiency, the options for taking a supplement may vary. You could take a supplement that has copper included with other vitamins and minerals or a supplement that is just copper. In some circumstances, copper is needed to aid in the absorption of other vitamins and minerals. For example, if a person has high levels of vitamin C or zinc, they may need more copper because vitamin C and zinc are known to interfere with the absorption of copper in the body.

If you do plan on taking any type of vitamin or mineral supplement, it is important to speak with your doctor before incorporating them into your daily regimen. A doctor can explain the proper way to take certain supplements as it relates to your personal health history and needs.[31]

Vitamins, Minerals, and Your Health

We need vitamins to regulate our cell function, organs, and overall development. Vitamins and minerals collectively help our eyes, heart, bones, joints, muscles, brain, mood, breathing, and so much more. Overall, they are needed for the body to function properly and keep us healthy.

Thirteen vitamins, called essential vitamins, are required for the body to have optimal function. The two categories of vitamins are fat-soluble and water-soluble. Fat-soluble vitamins are easily absorbed by the body and are stored in the liver, muscles, and fatty tissue. The fat-soluble vitamins are vitamins A, D, E, and K.

Water-soluble vitamins are not stored in the body and can be consumed through food or a supplement. Once a water-soluble vitamin is consumed, if there are any additional vitamins in the body that are not needed, it is released through urine. Water-soluble vitamins consist of all the B vitamins and vitamin C.[32]

The following is a list of all the essential vitamins:

º Biotin (vitamin B7)

31 "Office of Dietary Supplements—Copper," last updated October 18, 2022.

32 "Vitamins and Minerals," *National Center for Complementary and Integrative Health*, February 2018, https://www.nccih.nih.gov/health /vitamins-and-minerals.

- Cyanocobalamin (vitamin B12)
- Folate (vitamin B9)
- Niacin (vitamin B3)
- Pantothenic acid (vitamin B5)
- Pyridoxine (vitamin B6)
- Riboflavin (vitamin B2)
- Thiamine (vitamin B1)
- Vitamin A
- Vitamin C
- Vitamin D
- Vitamin E
- Vitamin K

The Benefits of Essential Vitamins

- **Vitamin A** aids in the development and sustainability of mucous membranes, skin, soft tissue, healthy teeth, and bones. Some foods that contain vitamin A are egg yolk, kale, broccoli, spinach, pumpkin, squash, sweet potatoes, tomatoes, dairy products, fish, beef, and liver.

- **Vitamin C** is a powerful antioxidant that helps the immune system fight against free radicals and aids in developing healthy gums, teeth, skin, and tissues. This vitamin also helps heal wounds and bruises. Some foods that contain vitamin C are oranges, grapefruits, kiwi, strawberries, tomatoes, potatoes, tomatoes, broccoli, and cruciferous vegetables such as brussels sprouts, cabbage, and cauliflower.

- **Vitamin D** is also known as the sunshine vitamin. It is recommended to get vitamin D through exposure to some natural sunlight around three times a week for about 15 minutes a day. If the sun is not a regular option, supplements may be required. Vitamin D is known to regulate the mood and absorb calcium, which helps strengthen bones and supports the immune system. Some foods that have this vitamin are egg yolk, beef liver, salmon, sardines, cod liver oil, tuna, fortified cereals, oatmeal, milk, yogurt, and orange juice.

o **Vitamin E** helps the brain, immune system, and skin. Containing antioxidant properties, vitamin E also forms healthy red blood cells, protects against free radicals, and assists with vision and reproduction. Some foods that contain vitamin E include mango, papaya, nuts, seeds, spinach, asparagus, turnip greens, broccoli, avocado, sunflower oil, and wheat germ.

o **Vitamin K** helps with proper bone function and blood function. Some foods that have vitamin K are spinach, kale, collard greens, turnip greens, broccoli, asparagus, fish, beef, liver, and eggs.

B Vitamins

o **Vitamin B2,** or riboflavin, is known to aid in maintaining the body's energy and helps to break down proteins, fats, and carbohydrates. This vitamin is also necessary to help the body produce healthy red blood cells and grow properly. Foods that have vitamin B2 include avocados, cayenne pepper, asparagus, dairy products, peas, molasses, mushrooms, parsley, pumpkin, and sage.

o **Vitamin B1,** or thiamine, helps the body break down glucose and creates energy metabolism from food. Other benefits include creating healthy brain function, healthy heart function, and regulating the nerves. Foods that have vitamin B1 include eggs, lean meats, legumes, nuts and seeds, peas, enriched bread, black beans, and acorn squash.

o **Vitamin B3,** or niacin, helps to maintain levels of HDL or high-density lipoprotein or what is commonly called "good" cholesterol. HDL helps with the removal of other forms of cholesterol from the body. Vitamin B3 also lowers triglycerides, which is a form of fat in the body that comes from animal fat and vegetable oil. Foods that have vitamin B3 are poultry, fish, avocado, legumes, eggs, and greens.

o **Vitamin B5,** or pantothenic acid, aids in the sustainability of metabolism. It also aids in producing healthy hormones and cholesterol. Some foods that have vitamin B5 are potatoes, organ meat, lentils, milk, kale, cabbage, broccoli, poultry, and mushrooms.

o **Vitamin B6,** or pyridoxine, converts food into energy. Vitamin B supports brain health, heart health, and the nervous system, and aids in the healthy production of red blood cells. Foods that have vitamin B6 are tuna, dark leafy green vegetables, salmon, chickpeas, bananas, cantaloupe, oranges, and beef liver.

o **Vitamin B7,** or biotin, helps the skin, hair, and overall health by regulating metabolism levels, regulating the heart, boosting immunity and brain function, and repairing the tissues and muscles. Foods that have vitamin B7 include beef liver, nuts, seeds, avocados, pork, sweet potatoes, and cooked eggs.

o **Vitamin B12,** or cyanocobalamin, helps to regulate the brain and nervous system, create DNA, and aid in the formation of healthy red blood cells. Vitamin B12 is in fish, dairy products, and meat.

o **Vitamin B9,** or folate, aids in forming healthy red blood cells and assists with cell growth and function. Vitamin B9 is important specifically for pregnant women because a folate deficiency can lead to birth defects. Vitamin B9 also helps the mental and emotional health of individuals. Foods that have vitamin B9 are lima beans, kidney beans, avocado, orange juice, salmon, turnips, beets, mustard greens, and root vegetables.[33]

Minerals and the Body

Just like vitamins, minerals are necessary to help the cells function normally in the body. There are two types of minerals: macrominerals and microminerals.

Macrominerals are minerals that are needed in large amounts. These minerals are calcium, chloride, magnesium, phosphorus, potassium, sodium, and sulfur. Some of the functions of macrominerals include the formation, growth, function, and repair of cells and bones.

○ **Calcium** is important for proper bone growth and protection. Calcium can help the formation of bones and teeth and sustain the strength of the body. Calcium can also help with the mobility of muscles, aid with blood flow, and sustain proper nerve functioning. Food sources of calcium include dairy products like cheese, milk, and yogurt; eggs; nut-based milk; kale; cabbage; spinach; and fatty fish.

○ **Chloride** helps to keep the blood pressure and PH levels in the body regulated. This mineral also is essential for regulating stomach fluids and carrying nerve impulses between the body and the brain. Foods that contain chloride are seaweed, tomatoes, lettuce, olives, and sea salt.

---

33 "Listing of Vitamins—Harvard Health," *Harvard Health*, August 31, 2020, https://www.health.harvard.edu/staying-healthy/listing_of_vitamins.

o **Magnesium** is a mineral that is found in the cells of your body. This mineral serves as a helper molecule, aiding in converting food into energy, muscle formation and mobility, nervous system regulation, protein creation from amino acids, and DNA and RNA creation and repair. The majority of magnesium in your body is in the bones. Other places are in the muscles, blood, and soft tissues. This mineral is also known to help with disease prevention. Health conditions that may be associated with low levels of magnesium include hypertension, type 2 diabetes, stroke, and migraines. Some food sources that include magnesium include spinach, white potatoes, whole grains, legumes, spinach, salmon, avocado, pumpkin seeds, bananas, and dark chocolate.[34]

o **Phosphorus** is the mineral that is responsible for the formation of teeth and bones. Approximately 85 percent of this mineral is stored in the teeth and bones. It also aids in the repair, growth, and sustainability of tissues and cells. This mineral also helps the body store energy by aiding the body in making adenosine triphosphate, or ATP, a molecule that is a source of energy for the cells, DNA, and RNA. Phosphorus helps regulate the heartbeat, normalize kidney function, signal nerves, and contract muscles. Some of the food sources that contain phosphorus are salmon, beef, yogurt, cheese, milk, legumes, poultry, tomatoes, asparagus, cauliflower, nuts, and seeds.[35]

---

34 Stella Lucia Volpe, "Magnesium in Disease Prevention and Overall Health," *Advances in Nutrition* 4, no. 3 (2013): 378S-383S, doi:10.3945/an .112.003483.

35 "Phosphorus," *The Nutrition Source*, accessed 28 August 2022, https:// www.hsph.harvard.edu/nutritionsource/phosphorus.

o **Potassium** helps deliver nutrients to the cells. It also aids in the proper function of the heart, muscles, and nerves. Some food sources for potassium include grapes, blackberries, carrots, spinach, grapefruit, oranges, and potatoes.[36]

o **Sodium** helps the body contract and relax muscles and conduct nerve impulses. Too much sodium can cause health conditions such as high blood pressure, stroke, and heart disease. Too much sodium can also cause calcium loss in the body.[37]

o **Sulfur** is a mineral that protects your cells from damage. It also aids in building and repairing the DNA. The amino acids methionine and cysteine in sulfur aid in making protein and the development and strengthening of skin, tendons, ligaments, hair, and nails. Sulfur is also present in biotin and thiamin. Some food sources of sulfur include eggs, chicken, beef, turkey, legumes, grains, lentils, walnuts, chickpeas, cabbage, kale, and radishes.[38]

Microminerals/Trace Minerals

Microminerals, also called trace minerals, are needed in smaller amounts. Although they are needed in small amounts they still play an important role in keeping the body healthy and functioning properly. Some of the functions of trace minerals include

---

36 "Office of Dietary Supplements—Potassium," National Institutes of Health, March 22, 2021, https://ods.od.nih.gov/factsheets/Potassium -Consumer.

37 "Salt and Sodium," *The Nutrition Source*, accessed August 28, 2022, https://www.hsph.harvard.edu/nutritionsource/salt-and-sodium.

38 Stephen Parcell, "Sulfur in Human Nutrition and Applications in Medicine," *Alternative Medicine Review* (2002), https://pubmed.ncbi.nlm.nih .gov/11896744.

supporting the blood system, aiding in normal growth, development, and neurological functions, proper hormone development, building enzymes, and protecting the body against free radicals. The major trace minerals or microminerals are chromium, copper fluoride, iodine, iron, manganese, and selenium.[39]

o **Copper** is a trace mineral that aids in keeping the nerve cells and immune system healthy. It also helps with producing red blood cells and collagen formation. The majority of copper is found in the heart, kidneys, skeletal muscle, brain, and liver. Some food sources of copper include almonds, beef liver, kale, oysters, salmon, spinach, sunflower seeds, cashews, avocado, and dark chocolate. There is more on foods and copper in Chapter Seven.

o **Chromium** is a trace mineral that improves the carbohydrate, lipid, and protein metabolism in the body. Some food sources of chromium include broccoli, potatoes, grape juice, and green beans.

o **Fluoride** is a mineral that is located in your teeth and bones. It also aids in preventing cavities. You can also find fluoride in water, plants, soil, rocks, and air. Fluoride is known to rebuild tooth enamel and help reverse tooth decay at the early stages. This mineral can be attained through water. Fluoride is known to be in a lot of dental items such as toothpaste and mouth rinses.

o **Iodine** is a mineral that the body doesn't make on its own. Iodine needs to be consumed through supplements and/ or food. The thyroid needs iodine to produce hormones that are needed for a healthy metabolism. Iodine also helps

---

39 "Minerals," Medline Plus, April 2, 2015, https://medlineplus.gov /minerals.html.

cognitive function. Individuals who are pregnant will also benefit from iodine because it helps the brain development of children. Once the babies are born, if breastfeeding is an option, the babies can continue to get iodine. Studies have shown that children with lower iodine levels have intellectual development issues. Some foods that have iodine include eggs, shrimp, tuna, and seaweed.

o **Iron** is a mineral that aids in the growth and development of the body. Iron helps the body make two proteins: myoglobin is a protein found in muscle tissue and hemoglobin is found in red blood cells. Iron is needed to help distribute red blood cells throughout the body. Iron also aids in helping the body make hormones. Iron also aids in sustaining energy and cognitive function in the body. Some of the food sources that contain iron include kidney beans, lentils, peas, lean meat, poultry, raisins, apricots, spinach, and iron-fortified bread and pasta.[40]

o **Manganese** helps metabolism, energy function, and digestion, and also has antioxidant properties that help to protect the body against free radicals. Another benefit includes bone development support. Foods that have manganese include mussels, hazelnuts, oysters, chickpeas, pecans, and brown rice.

o **Selenium** is a mineral that is essential for DNA production, healthy thyroid function, and protection from infection and free radicals. Some of the food sources that selenium

40 "Office of Dietary Supplements—Iron," National Institutes of Health, April 5, 2022, https://ods.od.nih.gov/factsheets/Iron-Consumer.

contains include Brazil nuts, cottage cheese, mushrooms, sunflower seeds, spinach, lentils, and bananas.[41]

Vitamin and Mineral and Deficiency

Many health conditions and illnesses can occur due to a vitamin and/or mineral deficiency. The type of illness depends specifically on the deficiency. Some of the health conditions that can occur due to vitamin and/or mineral deficiencies include:

- anemia
- depression
- weakened immune system
- tiredness
- nausea
- irregular heartbeat
- hair loss
- osteoporosis
- digestive issues
- numbness and tingling in different areas of the body
- poor appetite
- weakened connective tissue
- developmental issues in children
- brittle skin and nails
- skin discoloration
- lack of focus

If you have a deficiency, it is important to figure out why the deficiency is occurring, as the issue could be more than a lack of nutrition. Your primary care doctor or specialist can help you learn your levels and discuss options for your specific situation if you do have a deficiency in vitamins or minerals.

41 "Office of Dietary Supplements—Selenium," National Institutes of Health, March 22, 2022, https://ods.od.nih.gov/factsheets/Selenium-Consumer.

CHAPTER SEVEN

Copper and Food

There is nothing like a wonderful and delicious meal that serves the body with a plethora of natural vitamins and minerals. When we consistently eat healthy foods, we feel better naturally. There are some great foods that have copper, so it is not hard to get the necessary levels of copper through food.

The daily recommended intake of copper is fairly low at 900 mcg for both adult men and adult women. A balanced diet typically exceeds this amount of copper. The average amount of copper that is consumed through food is approximately 1,300 mcg for men and 1,100 mcg for women. When copper is consumed, it is primarily absorbed in the intestines and released by the liver. It goes into the bile to help protect the body from toxicity and copper deficiency.

As mentioned, it is very unlikely to consume too much copper through food. Overconsumption of copper typically occurs through mineral water or heavy metal and/or chemical exposure. If you are exposed to dust, air, or fumes that contain copper, it can enter the body and affect some organs including the lungs. In addition, there are some instances where water may have high levels of copper due to pipe erosion. If too much is consumed, copper toxicity can happen. More on copper toxicity is discussed later in the book.

Foods containing copper also have a lot of other vitamins and minerals that offer up great benefits for your overall health. I will list these on page 77.

So what does eating a healthy, nutrient-rich, and balanced diet actually mean?

A nutrient-dense diet consists of foods that are rich in nutrients, vitamins, and minerals. This includes fresh fruits and vegetables; nonfat and low-fat dairy; whole grains; fish and seafood; nuts; beans; legumes; lean, unprocessed meat; and poultry without the skin. It is also important to minimize and/or avoid heavily processed foods as well as unhealthy snacks that contain a lot of salt, sugar, and other additives that don't provide the body with proper nutrients to function properly. Consuming these foods long-term can cause health conditions and poor health.

Food and Energy

How much copper do we need? The body doesn't produce copper naturally. According to the Recommended Dietary Allowance (RDA), here is the amount of copper that is recommended for all ages. This is developed by the Food and Nutrition Board.[42]

---

42 "Office of Dietary Supplements—Copper," last updated October 18, 2022.

Table 1: Recommended Dietary Allowances (RDAs) for Copper**

Age	Male	Female	Pregnancy	Lactation
Birth to 6 months*	200 mcg	200 mcg		
7-12 months*	200 mcg	200 mcg		
1-3 years	340 mcg	340 mcg		
4-8 years	440 mcg	440 mcg		
9-13 years	700 mcg	700 mcg		
14-18 years	890 mcg	890 mcg	1,000 mcg	1,000 mcg
19+ years	900 mcg	900 mcg	1,300 mcg	1,300 mcg

*Adequate Intake (AI)
** Source: https://ods.od.nih.gov/factsheets/Copper-HealthProfessional

Foods That Have Copper

There are many delicious copper-friendly meal options for breakfast, lunch, and dinner. Here are some copper-enriched foods that are easy to incorporate into some of your meals.

Almonds

Almonds provide a wonderful source of antioxidants. Almonds are known to enhance the skin, support heart health, stabilize cholesterol levels, and help gut health with their high fiber content. In addition to copper, almonds contain vitamin E, magnesium, calcium, and protein.

You can add almonds to your diet by adding them to a smoothie, eating them alone, adding almonds to some fruit for granola, or adding them to a salad. Almonds are also a great addition to baked goods and oatmeal.

Avocado

Avocado is a fruit that has fat-soluble vitamins and a lot of wonderful benefits for the body. This fruit includes copper, folate, potassium, magnesium, beta carotene, protein, niacin, lutein, zeaxanthin, and omega fatty acids. Avocado also contains vitamins E, K, C, and B6. Avocado is known to aid in reducing cholesterol levels, help maintain weight, and reduce the risk of cardiovascular disease.[43] Avocado is also known to help eye health due to its zeaxanthin and lutein content. Some of the agents in avocados have antioxidant properties that offer protection to reduce damage from free radicals and UV lights. Nutrients in avocado may aid in reducing the risk of age-related macular degeneration. Due to its fiber content, it can also help regulate digestion.

You can add avocados to your diet by adding them to salads, sandwiches, toast, soups, eggs, and a wonderful guacamole recipe. Avocados can be a great substitute for sour cream and mayonnaise.[44]

Beef Liver

Beef liver comes from cattle. This food is a micronutrient with a lot of vitamins and minerals. Along with copper, beef liver has vitamins A, B12, B6, iron, pantothenic acid, riboflavin, phosphorus, zinc, thiamin, manganese, niacin, and selenium. Beef liver is

---

43 Patrícia Fonseca Duarte et al., "Avocado: Characteristics, Health Benefits and Uses," *Ciência Rural* 46, no. 4 (2016): 747–754, doi:10.1590/0103-8478 cr20141516.

44 Tammy Scott et al., "Avocado Consumption Increases Macular Pigment Density in Older Adults: A Randomized, Controlled Trial," *Nutrients* 9, no. 9 (2017): 919, doi:10.3390/nu9090919.

known to help people with anemia due to the high levels of B12 and iron. This food also helps with oxygen distribution in the body and aids in keeping the immune system healthy. Although beef liver is full of wonderful vitamins and minerals, too much consumption of beef liver can lead to vitamin A toxicity. Beef liver can be prepared as a great lunch and dinner option.

You add beef liver to your diet by mixing it with onions and eating it with vegetables or rice. Avoid overcooking beef liver so it can stay tender.[45]

Cassava

A root that originates in South America, cassava has a lot of nutrients and vitamins that help the overall health of the body. This root is also known as yucca and has a texture that is similar to the potato when it is cooked. Some of the many vitamins and minerals that cassava root has include fiber, vitamin C, thiamine, niacin, potassium, vitamin B6, folate, magnesium, and antioxidants. Cassava root is known to improve immunity, support collagen production, aid in neurotransmitter synthesis and energy production, support iron metabolism, and protect the body against free radicals. It is also known to normalize blood pressure and enhance the tone and elasticity of the skin.

You can add cassava to your diet by preparing it similarly to mashed potatoes.[46]

45 "Office of Dietary Supplements—Iron," National Institutes of Health, April 5, 2022, https://ods.od.nih.gov/factsheets/Iron-Consumer.

46 Pingjuan Zhao et al., "Analysis of Different Strategies Adapted by Two Cassava Cultivars in Response to Drought Stress: Ensuring Survival or Continuing Growth," *Journal of Experimental Botany* 66, no. 5 (2014): 1477–1488, doi:10.1093/jxb/eru507.

Chia Seeds

Chia seeds are a flowering plant from the mint family. The seeds are native to the South American region. These seeds have a lot of antioxidants, vitamins, and minerals. Along with protein, chia seeds are also known to have omega-three fatty acids. Some of the health benefits include reducing free radicals, improving heart health, and lowering high blood pressure. Chia seeds can also improve blood sugar levels and reduce inflammation in the body. Due to the high fiber content, they are known to help intestinal health. Chia seeds also have calcium and help sustain bone health. They are also known to help with weight management due to the fact that they help you feel full longer when consumed.

Consuming chia seeds is easy since they are tasteless.

You can add chia seeds to your diet by putting them in your oatmeal, smoothie, or salad. You can also add them to your power balls or homemade energy bars. Chia seed pudding is also a great meal or snack option to eat and enjoy.[47]

Dark Chocolate

Dark chocolate is a great option for an occasional treat. Although we shouldn't indulge in it, it does have lower sugar and fat content than milk chocolate. Dark chocolate is also known to have a lot of antioxidants. Although there is sugar in dark chocolate, there is less sugar added because there is about 50 percent to 90 percent of cocoa in dark chocolate. This food is known to

47 Rahman Ullah et al., "Nutritional and Therapeutic Perspectives of Chia (Salvia Hispanica L.): A Review," *Journal of Food Science and Technology* 53, no. 4 (2015): 1750–1758, doi:10.1007/s13197-015-1967-0.

help relax your blood vessels and aid in lowering blood pressure. Dark chocolate has a lot of minerals such as zinc, copper, phosphorus, fiber, and magnesium, which can help you sleep. It may be associated with increasing your mood due to some of the antioxidant agents that are in the food. Dark chocolate is a great alternative to satisfy a sweet tooth as a healthier option.

You can add dark chocolate to your diet by enjoying the occasional dark chocolate bar.[48]

Kale

Kale is a member of the cabbage family with vitamins A, C, B6, and K. It also has magnesium, copper, protein, potassium, beta carotene, and antioxidants. Kale is known to be a very nutridense food. Due to many of the properties in kale, this vegetable is known to aid in lowering blood pressure, reducing high cholesterol, and helping with eye health.

You can add kale to your diet by eating it as a salad, adding it to your smoothies, adding it as an ingredient in fresh juice, or cooking it with other vegetables such as collard greens and cabbage.[49]

---

48 María Ángeles Martin and Sonia Ramos, "Impact of Cocoa Flavanols on Human Health," *Food and Chemical Toxicology* 151 (2021): 112121, doi:10.1016/j.fct.2021.112121.

49 Elżbieta Sikora and Izabela Bodziarczyk, "Composition and Antioxidant Activity of Kale (Brassica Oleracea L. Var. Acephala) Raw and Cooked," *Acta Scientiarum Polonorum Technologia Alimentaria* 11, no. 3 (2012): 239–248, https://pubmed.ncbi.nlm.nih.gov/22744944.

Kidney Beans

Kidney beans have a lot of wonderful health benefits. They offer protein, which is helpful for those on a plant-based diet. Along with copper, kidney beans also offer folate, magnesium, potassium, vitamins E, K, and B1, and iron. Kidney beans give you energy and aid in memory function due to the vitamin B1 components. It also aids in regulating and lowering cholesterol levels. Other benefits include anti-aging properties due to the antioxidants, helping bone health due to the magnesium, and reducing inflammation due to the fiber. This bean can also aid in weight loss.[50] In a study of thirty obese adults, findings showed that eating beans approximately four times a week had a greater weight-loss effect than consuming a bean-free diet. Another benefit is that they contain a class of lectin that is known to block and/or delay the absorption of carbohydrates from the diet. Although overconsumption of beans can cause bloating and gas, it can be a delicious option to add to your diet.[51]

You can add kidney beans to salad, soup, rice, or pasta. You can also create a bean dip or eat them as a side dish.

Lentils

Lentils come from the grain family in different colors. You may see them in brown, green, yellow, red, or beluga, which is also black. Lentils are a very nutritious food. Along with copper,

---

50 Wokadala Cuthbert Obiro, Tao Zhang and Bo Jiang, "The Nutraceutical Role of Thephaseolus Vulgarisa-Amylase Inhibitor," *British Journal of Nutrition* 100, no. 1 (2008): 1–12, doi:10.1017/s0007114508879135.

51 Paul K. Whelton and Jiang He, "Health Effects of Sodium and Potassium in Humans," *Current Opinion in Lipidology* 25, no. 1 (2014): 75–79, doi:10.1097/mol.0000000000000033.

lentils have potassium, zinc, magnesium, vitamin B, and pro-tein.[52] This is a great food as a meat alternative for people who consume a plant-based diet. Lentils are also a great source of iron, fiber, thiamine, folate, magnesium, phosphorus, potassium, zinc, and manganese. Lentils offer wonderful anti-inflammatory benefits due to their strong antioxidant agents. This food can also aid in reducing heart disease, diabetes, high cholesterol levels, and obesity. A study with thirty-nine participants who were overweight consumed 60 grams of lentils each day. This is equivalent to approximately a third of a cup. The results showed a reduction in their cholesterol levels.[53]

To add lentils to your diet, you can make soup, lentil burgers, or add them to vegetables or rice.

Mango

Mango is a sweet fruit that is enjoyed throughout the world. Some of the vitamins and minerals that mango has along with copper include fiber, copper, folate, vitamins C, B6, E, A, and K. Mangos also have potassium, riboflavin, thymine, and mag-nesium. Mango helps with the growth and development of the body, improves the appearance of the skin, aids in digestive health, helps heart health, and helps the immune system.

To add mangos to your diet, enjoy them as a snack or dessert. You can eat them alone, add them to your smoothies, oatmeal,

52 Kumar Ganesan and Baojun Xu, "Polyphenol-Rich Lentils and Their Health Promoting Effects," *International Journal of Molecular Sciences* 18, no. 11 (2017): 2390, doi:10.3390/ijms18112390.

53 Zahra Aslani et al., "Lentil Sprouts Effect on Serum Lipids of Overweight and Obese Patients With Type 2 Diabetes," *Health Promotion Perspectives* 5, no. 3 (2015): 215–224, doi:10.15171/hpp.2015.026.

and yogurt, or make a fruit salad. You can also make a mango-based salsa or add it to a leafy green salad.[54]

Oysters

Along with copper, oysters have potassium, vitamins D and B12, iron, phosphorus, zinc, manganese, and selenium. Some of the health benefits of oysters include increasing energy levels, strengthening the immune system, and sustaining blood levels. Oysters are also known to aid in the reduction of osteoporosis symptoms. Although people either love or dislike oysters, there are also some who may be allergic. If you are not sure if you are allergic to oysters, have a conversation with your doctor.[55]

To add oysters to your diet, enjoy them alone or with a meal.

Pomegranates

Pomegranates are a fruit that offers a plethora of antioxidants and anti-inflammatory compounds. This fruit is known to help with urinary, brain, digestive, and prostate health. Pomegranates are also known to aid in fighting off bacteria, yeast, and fungi in the body. In addition, the fruit helps the urinary tract by reducing the formation of kidney stones. There are studies that report that pomegranate juice helps reduce inflammation in

---

54 Veeranjaneya Reddy Lebaka et al., "Nutritional Composition and Bioactive Compounds in Three Different Parts of Mango Fruit," *International Journal of Environmental Research and Public Health* 18, no. 2 (2021): 741, doi:10.3390/ijerph18020741.

55 Fumio Watanabe et al., "Characterization of Vitamin B 12 Compounds from Edible Shellfish, Clam, Oyster, and Mussel," *International Journal of Food Sciences and Nutrition* 52, no. 3 (2001): 263–268, doi:10.1080/0963748 0020027000-3-6.

humans. Along with copper, pomegranate has protein, calcium, iron, folate, antioxidants, potassium, and magnesium.

Pomegranate is a wonderful fruit to enjoy on its own as well as in fresh juices and smoothies.[56]

Quinoa

Though it has been around since ancient times, quinoa has recently gained in popularity. Quinoa is very nutrient dense, and it has a lot of essential vitamins and minerals. Along with copper, this food has fiber, folate, vitamins B6 and E, iron, magnesium, phosphorus, and potassium. Many appreciate this food's high protein content and amino acids. In addition, quinoa has high levels of antioxidants. Quinoa aids in reducing inflammation, regulating blood sugar, and regulating weight. This food will help you feel full longer due to its heavy nutrient content.

Enjoy quinoa in a salad, in a breakfast smoothie or oatmeal, or as an addition to a wonderful power bowl for dinner. Quinoa is also a great food used in place of a carbohydrate.[57]

Salmon

Salmon is a great fish to create many recipes. It also has a lot of vitamins and minerals that can lead to wonderful health benefits. Along with containing copper, salmon is a fatty fish that offers protein, selenium, vitamin B, vitamin D, phosphorus, omega-

---

56 Vesna Vučić et al., "Composition and Potential Health Benefits of Pomegranate: A Review," *Current Pharmaceutical Design* 25, no. 16 (2019): 1817–1827, doi:10.2174/1381612825666190708183941.

57 Eng Shi Ong et al., "Antioxidant and Cytoprotective Effect of Quinoa (Chenopodium Quinoa Willd.) with Pressurized Hot Water Extraction (PHWE)," *Antioxidants* 9, no. 11 (2020): 1110, doi:10.3390/antiox9111110.

three fatty acids, and more. Salmon is known to help nerve function, reduce inflammation in the body, help your brain, aid in normalizing and reducing blood pressure, help muscle function, vision, and bone health. Due to its antioxidant properties, salmon is known to reduce the levels of bad cholesterol.

There are many ways that you can incorporate salmon into your diet. You can eat it in a salad, enjoy it alongside vegetables, and/or scramble it with some eggs for breakfast.[58]

Spinach

Spinach is a potent vegetable that offers a lot of vitamins, minerals, and health benefits.

In addition to copper it also has protein, fiber, folic acid, calcium, vitamin C, and vitamin A. Spinach also has iron, a mineral that aids in creating hemoglobin, which helps brings oxygen to the tissues of the body. Consuming spinach also aids in the maintenance of bone health. Spinach also helps the immune system and the appearance of the skin. Due to its antioxidant properties, spinach helps the body protect itself from free radicals and oxidative stress.

To include spinach in your diet, you can eat spinach salads, add it to other leafy greens, or sauté spinach as a side dish. Spinach can also be juiced and added to a smoothie. This vegetable can be cooked with other items such as eggs and pasta, or added to a delicious power bowl.[59]

58 "Fish: Friend Or Foe?" *The Nutrition Source*, accessed August 28, 2022, https://www.hsph.harvard.edu/nutritionsource/fish.

59 "Spinach," *Nutrition Data*, accessed August 28, 2022, https://nutritiondata.self.com/facts/vegetables-and-vegetable-products/2626/2.

Spirulina

Spirulina grows in saltwater and freshwater. It is also referred to as blue-green algae. This food has vitamins and minerals such as copper, protein, vitamins B1, B2, and B3, iron, and omega-3 and omega-6 fatty acids. Due to the high level of antioxidant properties, it also has anti-inflammatory benefits that aid in preventing oxidative damage in the body. Spirulina can help keep the immune system healthy, protect the body from oxidation, ease indigestion, and aid in heart health, diabetes, and maintaining healthy cholesterol levels. A study of 25 participants with type 2 diabetes took 2 grams of spirulina each day for two months. The results showed that both the postprandial, the glucose level in the body after eating a meal, and fasting blood glucose levels were lower.

Spirulina can be consumed as a supplement. It can also be added to a smoothie, water, and/or juice.[60]

Shiitake Mushrooms

Shiitake mushrooms are known for their savory taste and are a popular mushroom to add to recipes. Native to East Asia, these mushrooms are also grown in Japan. Other countries that produce them are Canada, Singapore, China, and the United States. Some of the many vitamins and minerals that shiitake mushrooms contain along with copper include protein, fiber, niacin, zinc, vitamins B5, B6, and D, manganese, zinc, and selenium. Some of the health benefits of shiitake mushrooms

---

60 Eun Hee Lee et al., "A Randomized Study to Establish the Effects of Spirulina in Type 2 Diabetes Mellitus Patients," *Nutrition Research and Practice* 2, no. 4 (2008): 295, doi:10.4162/nrp.2008.2.4.295.

include aiding in intestinal health and nerve function, keeping the immune system healthy, aiding in heart health, and protecting the bones.

Shiitake mushrooms have strong consistency and they are great in stir-fry, vegetable dishes, or with a sautéed meat such as beef or chicken.[61]

Sweet Potatoes

Sweet potatoes are a staple for the holiday table. One item that comes to mind is sweet potato pie. This vegetable has wonderful benefits that will keep you healthy throughout the year. There are different colors to sweet potatoes, the most familiar being orange. You may also see purple, white, or a yellowish hue. Some of the many vitamins and minerals that sweet potatoes have alongside copper include vitamins A, C, and B6, manganese, potassium, fiber, and niacin. Sweet potatoes also have a lot of antioxidants. Sweet potatoes can help the body protect itself against free radicals, aid in eye health, and reduce inflammation. Sweet potatoes also aid in supporting gut health, brain health, and the nervous and immune systems.

61 Yearul Kabir, Mami Yamaguchi, and Shuichi Kimura, "Effect of Shiitake (Lentinus Edodes) and Maitake(Grifola Frondosa) Mushrooms on Blood Pressure and Plasma Lipids of Spontaneously Hypertensive Rats," *Journal of Nutritional Science and Vitaminology* 33, no. 5 (1987): 341–346, doi:10.3177/jnsv.33.341.

Sweet potatoes can be added to your breakfast instead of white potatoes. You can also create baked sweet potatoes, make a soup, sauté them, and make sweet potato fries.[62]

Turnip Greens

Turnip greens are a cruciferous vegetable with many health benefits. Some of the vitamins and minerals that turnip greens have along with copper include folate, magnesium, potassium, vitamins C and K, calcium, and phosphorus. Turnip greens also have antioxidants. The health benefits of turnip greens include reducing the risk of high blood pressure, kidney stones, high blood sugar, stroke, and brittle bones. Turnip greens are also known to help keep red blood cells healthy.

You can incorporate turnip greens into your diet by eating them for lunch or dinner, steaming the greens with other vegetables, or adding them to soups.[63]

With all of the delicious copper-containing food options that also contain a plethora of vitamins and minerals, the body will truly benefit. It is important to remember that moderation and balance are key when eating any type of food.

---

62 Xin Wang et al., "The Inhibitory Effects of Purple Sweet Potato Color on Hepatic Inflammation Is Associated With Restoration of NAD+ Levels and Attenuation of NLRP3 Inflammasome Activation in High-Fat-Diet-Treated Mice," *Molecules* 22, no. 8 (2017): 1315, doi:10.3390/molecules22081315.

63 "Turnips, Raw," *Food Data Central*, accessed August 28, 2022, https://fdc .nal.usda.gov/fdc-app.html#/food-details/170465/nutrients.

CHAPTER EIGHT

Copper and Supplements

Every day, many people reach for some type of vitamin or mineral supplement in the morning before they get their day started. Others take their vitamins at night. The reasons why they take supplements may vary. Some could be taking the suggestion of their doctor. Others may be acting in self-interest to ensure they are getting what they need to stay healthy. Still, others may have a specific condition that requires supplementation. There are a lot of options when it comes to vitamins, minerals, and herbal supplements. This short chapter discusses supplements and their benefits in general.

It is important to try to get your vitamins and minerals through foods. This is not possible for everyone, so do the best you can to keep your body healthy and nourished. While there are times when processed foods are the easiest and only options, these foods do have limited nutritional value.

Processed foods also contain many of chemicals and may give you a false sense of satiation without providing the nutrients needed to stay healthy. Consuming highly processed foods long term is known to cause health conditions as well as vitamin and mineral deficiencies. In addition to processed foods, certain medications can also cause a vitamin and mineral deficiency.[64]

Taking dietary supplements is not uncommon. Many people turn to vitamins, or minerals, or herbal supplements to make sure they are getting all of the vitamins and minerals necessary to keep the body functioning properly. In the United States alone, multivitamins and multimineral supplements are taken by approximately one-third of adults and one-quarter of children and adolescents.[65]

Reasons why people may take supplements include the following:

o Dietary intake to make sure they are getting enough quantities of vitamins and minerals if the food they consume does not.

o Illness prevention. The common cold can be avoided with vitamins and minerals such as vitamin C, zinc, and vitamin D to boost immune function.

o Other health conditions. Those with certain illnesses may experience side effects from their medication. Long-term use of medications can cause an interference with the body's ability to absorb and/or produce nutrients.

Studies show that people who take multivitamin or mineral supplements have higher micronutrient levels in their body. A large number of micronutrients are not required to help the body func-

64 "Should You Take Dietary Supplements? A Look at Vitamins, Minerals, Botanicals, and More," National Institutes of Health, 2013, https://newsinhealth.nih.gov/2013/08/should-you-take-dietary-supplements.

65 "Office of Dietary Supplements—Multivitamin/Mineral Supplements," National Institutes of Health, 2022, https://ods.od.nih.gov/factsheets/MVMS-HealthProfessional.

tion properly; they are also not consumed enough through food alone. It takes conscious effort to incorporate the foods that will give the proper amount of micronutrients. If there is a minimal deficiency, supplements can help you get the proper amount of micronutrients that are needed in the body.[66] One micronutrient that is needed to ensure the body functions properly is copper.

Copper Supplements

If you don't have the proper levels of copper in your body, you can adjust your diet to eat foods that have copper, or you can take a supplement.

There are some cases when a copper supplement is necessary and/or a series of supplements should be taken to help the body absorb copper and other vitamins and minerals.

For example, a common sign of copper deficiency is anemia. Although anemia is due to low iron consumption, low levels of copper can cause anemia as well. Studies show that copper has the potential to interfere with iron absorption. This happens when copper binds to the mucosal transferrin, a blood-plasma glycoprotein that is responsible for the iron metabolism.

Another mineral that can reduce the absorption of copper is zinc. If a zinc supplement is taken in high levels for a long period of time, it is known to cause a copper deficiency. It is also common for people with osteoporosis to have low copper levels in the body. Some individuals may have acquired and

---

66 "Office of Dietary Supplements—Multivitamin/Mineral Supplements," National Institutes of Health, June 22, 2022, https://ods.od.nih.gov /factsheets/MVMS-Consumer.

inherited copper deficiency, which may require supplementation. In addition, high levels of vitamin C can also interfere with copper absorption.

Many multivitamins and minerals have copper included in them, and this could be enough to get the levels of copper needed to satisfy the daily recommended requirement and help sustain levels of other vitamins and minerals in the body. Some situations require a copper supplement alone. If you do need copper supplementation, your doctor can help you determine what you need specifically.[67]

There are different forms of copper supplements: those formed with other binding ingredients, pure copper supplements, and multivitamins that include copper along with other vitamins, minerals, and ingredients. There are also different forms of copper that are in the supplements and serve to control bacteria. These include copper amino acid chelates, copper gluconate, a blue green crystal or powder that is taken for a copper deficiency, cupric oxide, an antimicrobial used in food production and in some pharmaceuticals, and cupric sulfate, which is known to control the fungus and bacteria on fruits and vegetables. One of the most common types of copper used is chelated. This form is bound to a protein molecule or an amino acid to make it easier for absorption in the body.

Copper supplements can come in pill and liquid forms. It is important that you work closely with your doctor to avoid consuming too much copper as well. As mentioned on page 47 and page 48, copper toxicity can lead to illness, severe headaches, diarrhea, vomiting, metallic taste in the mouth, stomach

---

67 "Copper," *Linus Pauling Institute*, accessed August 28, 2022, https://lpi .oregonstate.edu/mic/minerals/copper.

pain, dizziness, and in extreme cases, heart complications, jaundice, and abnormal formation of the red blood cells.

CHAPTER NINE

Copper and the Immune System

As the body's natural defense system, the immune system protects the body from infections caused by intruders like viruses, fungi, parasites, and bacteria that can invade the body and cause illnesses. Proper diet, exercise, sleep, and reduced stress are some of the ways to keep the immune system strong. When the immune system can't fully protect the body, medication and other treatments will assist in fighting off infection and germs or pathogens.

Copper helps the development and maintenance of the immune system. When copper levels are low in the body, it becomes a challenge to make immune cells and that can lead to a low white blood cell count. In order to keep the immune system healthy, it is important to understand some of the elements that make up the immune system and help it function properly.

First is the analysis of some of the elements that make up the immune system. For example, cytokines. These are proteins that are produced by cells. Cytokines are known to aid in regulating the body's response to infection and disease. They also normalize the cellular process in the body. Another example is leukocytes.

97

These are white blood cells that help the body fight infection.[68] White blood cells come from the bone marrow and lymphatic tissues. They help fight infection by increasing the cell defense against infection in the body, blood infection, and some other illnesses and disorders that may occur. Antibodies, also known as immunoglobulin, are another example. These are proteins produced by the immune system that protects the body from disease and infection. This shows the overview and overall health of the immune system.

The second approach is to look at the functionality of the immune system and analyze how well it fights off infection and disease overall. If some areas of the immune system are lacking, this could be due to vitamin and mineral deficiencies and/or diseases within the body. The third approach is how the immune system responds to any challenges that the body may face when disease, infection, and/or illness occurs. Copper helps the body by maintaining the health of the immune system.[69]

When it comes to keeping the immune system healthy, the common thought that may come to mind is to do your part to stay healthy. Others focus on keeping the immune system healthy by increasing their intake of vitamins, minerals, and herbal supplements. Taking the right steps to keep your immune system healthy can lead to confidence in knowing that you are doing your part to protect yourself against major and minor illnesses.

68 "Overview of the Immune System," National Institute of Allergy and Infections Diseases, 2022, https://www.niaid.nih.gov/research/immune-system-overview.

69 "The Immune System," John Hopkins Medicine, 2022, https://www.hopkinsmedicine.org/health/conditions-and-diseases/the-immune-system.

As the seasons change and the common cold and flu are more common, many people become more conscious of their vitamin and mineral intake so they can stay healthy all year. In addition, more people are strongly rethinking how the immune system works and what they can do on a daily basis to stay healthy and keep their immune systems healthy and strong.

The Function of the Immune System

If an illness occurs and the immune system is healthy and functioning well, it can do one of two things: block the illness from entering the body, or if the illness occurs, reduce the symptoms. This is all dependent on the specific illness and person. Everyone has a different reaction to illness and their own body chemistry makeup.

There are situations where people have illnesses such as cancer, HIV, diabetes, multiple sclerosis, and other autoimmune diseases that can naturally weaken the immune system. This can make it difficult for the person to fight off additional illnesses. In addition, if a person has an illness and takes medication for that specific illness, some side effects of the medication are known to reduce the strength of the immune system. This can make it more difficult to fight off infection. If a person has a vitamin and/or mineral deficiencies, the immune system may not function at its full capacity.

Some of the top tips for keeping the immune system healthy include eating a healthy diet, staying hydrated, reducing the consumption of foods that have high amounts of sugar and salt, avoiding highly processed foods, and washing your body and hands regularly as well as keeping the area where you spend a lot of your time clean, such as your home, car, and workstations.[70]

Other tips include getting proper rest, staying hydrated, exercising regularly, keeping your stress levels low, and minimizing the use of alcohol and tobacco.

Once you find your flow with creating a healthy lifestyle, you naturally feel good. When you are feeling good and healthy, the immune system and its functionality is probably not top of mind. Typically, it is when we get sick or encounter an illness that may require time to heal when we think about the immune system and its purpose. Naturally, we also think about getting better and the things we need to do to sustain our health and wellness.

Immune System Makeup

There are two major parts to your immune system: the innate immune system and the adaptive immune system. They work together to help protect the body. You are born with an innate immune system. It consists of the cornea of the eye, the skin, and the mucous membranes that line the genitourinary, gastrointestinal, and respiratory tracts. When a virus or bacteria tries to enter the body, the innate immune system recognizes the bacte-

---

70 "How to Boost Your Immune System—Harvard Health," *Harvard Health*, February 15, 2021, https://www.health.harvard.edu/staying-healthy/how-to -boost-your-immune-system.

ria and acts immediately to help the body fight off any infection or virus that tries to threaten the body.[71]

The adaptive immune system, also called the active immune system, works with the innate immune system. The adaptive immune system initially doesn't move as quickly as the innate immune system. The adaptive immune system is known to work from its memory system. Once a germ enters the body, the adaptive immune system remembers it. When that specific germ enters the body again, it will react faster and try to protect the body against the specific germ and then will react faster to fight the bacteria. This helps to fight off infection because it remembers the germs that have previously entered the body.

In the event that the innate immune system doesn't respond, the adaptive immune system will take over and help the body fight infection.

Along with the innate and adaptive immune systems, there are a collection of cells and organs that are also included in the immune system. These include the following:

- Bone marrow
- Lymphatic system
- Mucous membranes
- Skin
- Spleen
- Stomach
- Tonsils
- Thymus
- White blood cells

---

71 "The Innate and Adaptive Immune Systems," National Institutes of Health, July 30, 2020, https://www.ncbi.nlm.nih.gov/books/NBK279396.

Bone Marrow

The majority of the cells that are part of the immune system are produced in the bone marrow. Once the immune system cells are produced, they multiply. The bone marrow also creates new blood cells daily and feeds them into your bloodstream. This is also the area where white blood cells and plasma are produced. Initially, when we are born, the majority of bones have red bone marrow, and this creates immune system cells. As we age, the bone marrow turns into fatty tissue and the only bones that still have red bone marrow are the pelvis, breastbone, and ribs.

Lymphatic System

The lymph nodes are immune cells that help to destroy and prevent germs from going to other parts of your body and causing illness. Once the lymph node identifies the bacteria, they send the white blood cells to help fight the bacteria that enter the body. The lymphatic system has the ability to deliver nutrients to the cells. This happens with the organs and tissues that are a part of the lymphatic system. Collectively these organs, vessels, and tissues help to maintain healthy blood flow and create and sustain a healthy immune system. The lymphatic system consists of the lymph, collecting ducts, lymph nodes, and lymphatic vessels. Some of the major functions of the lymphatic system include protecting the body against germs, bacteria, and viruses. It recirculates fluid levels throughout the body; serves as a filter and removes abnormal cells and waste; and releases white blood cells and other cells aligned with immune function to help fight bacteria, fungi, parasites, and viruses.[72]

Mucous Membranes

These membranes protect the body against germs in several ways. As the mucous membranes secrete mucus, there are times when germs enter the body and try to stick to the mucus. This is a way that infection can enter the body. In order to prevent the infection from entering the body and spreading, the tiny hairs, also known as the cilia, help to move the germs out of the area where they are trying to invade the body. Other portions of the mucous membranes that protect the body against germs are the enzymes that are in tears, sweat, and secretions in the vagina.

Skin

The skin is the largest organ in the body and helps the body protect itself against germs with natural oils and the secretion of immune system cells.[73]

Spleen

The spleen is located above your stomach and is in the left rib cage. Although it is a small organ, it has an important and impactful role in the body. Some of the functions of the spleen include filtering blood and getting rid of damaged and old blood

---

72 Shan Liao and Timothy P. Padera, "Lymphatic Function and Immune Regulation in Health and Disease," *Lymphatic Research and Biology* 11, no. 3 (2013): 136–143, doi:10.1089/lrb.2013.0012.

73 "What Are the Organs of the Immune System?," National Institutes of Health, July 30, 2020, https://www.ncbi.nlm.nih.gov/books/NBK279395/#_NBK279395_pubdet.

cells. The spleen also stores blood and maintains healthy levels of fluids. This organ also creates white blood cells and antibodies, which helps protect the body against infection. The spleen has two parts: the red pulp and the white pulp. The red pulp destroys bacteria and viruses. It also removes waste from the blood, getting rid of damaged and old blood cells. The other part of the spleen is the white pulp. This is the area that is part of the immune system. The white pulp produces white blood cells. The white blood cells make antibodies.[74]

Stomach

The stomach is part of the gastrointestinal tract, which is an important part of the digestive system. The stomach produces digestive juices and the chemical reaction that helps to break down the food to move into the small intestine. The three main functions of the stomach are to store food, break the food down, and produce enzymes so the food can properly digest in the body.

The acid in the stomach can help kill the bacteria after it enters your body. There are also good bacteria that eliminate the harmful bacteria that can make you ill. Seventy to 80 percent of immune cells are known to be present in the gut. When your gut is healthy, your stomach and intestines can function properly and aid in reducing infection in the body.[75]

---

74 Vaishali Kapila, Chase Wehrle and Faiz Tuma, "Physiology, Spleen," National Institutes of Health, May 8, 2022, https://www.ncbi.nlm.nih.gov /books/NBK537307.

75 Selma P. Wiertsema et al., "The Interplay Between the Gut Microbiome and the Immune System in the Context of Infectious Diseases Throughout Life and the Role of Nutrition in Optimizing Treatment Strategies," *Nutrients* 13, no. 3 (2021): 886, doi:10.3390/nu13030886.

Tonsils

The tonsils can help stop bacteria from entering the body through the nose or mouth. This organ also has a lot of white blood cells. These cells are instrumental in killing germs. There are three types of tonsils that collectively help protect the body: the palatine, the adenoids, and the lingual tonsil. The tonsils also have cells that produce antibodies. The antibodies can help prevent the body from getting germs that can lead to infections of the throat and lungs.[76]

Thymus

The thymus is a small organ that makes and produces T-lymphocyte, or T-cells. These are white blood cells that originate in the bone marrow. T-cells are an important function of the immune system as they help to fight off infection. The thymus is located beneath the breastbone in the upper area of the chest. This organ protects against tumors, antigens, and pathogens. This organ also helps the body protect against infection because it remembers invasive germs in the body. Once the germs enter the body, the thymus goes into protection mode to prevent their attempt spread infection and create illness.

White Blood Cells

White blood cells are one of the most important parts of your immune system. Also known as leukocytes, the white blood cells are located in the bloodstream and travel throughout the tissues and blood vessel walls. They produce antibody proteins to help

---

76 "How Do the Tonsils Work?," National Library of Medicine, January 17, 2019, https://www.ncbi.nlm.nih.gov/books/NBK279406.

destroy the bacteria, viruses, and infections. White blood cells are formed within the soft tissue of the bone marrow. White blood cells respond to injury, bacteria, or illness by circulating in the blood. As one white blood cell identifies a possible threat or infection to the body, other white blood cells join together to help the body fight off the infection.[77]

Vitamins and Minerals and the Immune System

When there is a lack of nutrition in the body, this can lead to a lack of energy, illness, and a lot of deficiencies in the micronutrients that are needed to keep the immune function healthy. Deficiencies in the vitamins and minerals can cause negative impacts on the immune system. With a weakened immune system, the body can't fight off infection effectively.

There are some specific vitamins and minerals that aid in keeping the immune system healthy. These vitamins and minerals include but are not limited to copper, folic acid, iron, selenium, vitamin A, vitamin B complex, vitamin C, vitamin D, vitamin E, and zinc.[78] It is important to get your daily recommended values of all of the vitamins and minerals (see page 64) so your body can stay healthy.

---

77 "Hematology Glossary," Hematology.org, accessed August 29, 2022, https://www.hematology.org/education/patients/blood-basics.

78 Adrian F. Gombart, Adeline Pierre and Silvia Maggini, "A Review of Micronutrients and the Immune System–Working in Harmony to Reduce the Risk of Infection," *Nutrients* 12, no. 1 (2020): 236, doi:10.3390/nu12010236.

Copper and the Immune System

Although the specifics of how copper is involved in the immune system are not clearly defined, it does have an effect on immune health. Copper has antioxidant properties and enzymes. Two enzymes that are dependent on copper are superoxide dismutase and ceruloplasmin. Both of these enzymes have anti-inflammatory abilities. They also prevent tissue damage due to inflammation and infection.

In addition, research shows that there is a strong connection between the immune responsiveness of T-cells and copper. One of the diagnoses of copper deficiency is neutropenia. One of the symptoms of this condition is extremely low levels of white blood cells. When the white blood cells are low and/or not functioning properly, the immune system can't function at its highest capacity. When there is a copper deficiency, research shows that the immune systems are compromised. This can range from infants and children who have Menkes disease, a genetic disorder with symptoms of an extreme copper deficiency, to adults who have low levels of white blood cells due to a copper deficiency.[79]

Some factors that can weaken the immune system are the following:

Environment

There are specific industries where the body is exposed to toxins. Depending on where you live and what type of work you do, this can include but is not limited to smoke, air pollution, and industry-specific toxins that can damage the immune system and

---

79 Maxine Bonham et al., "The Immune System as a Physiological Indicator of Marginal Copper Status?," *British Journal of Nutrition* 87, no. 5 (2002): 393–403, doi:10.1079/BJN2002558.

other organs after an extended amount of exposure. If you do spend time around chemicals and equipment that is toxic or may have the potential to be harmful after long-term use, contact your doctor. They can help you get tested to see if the substances that you are exposed to influence your health short and long term.

Obesity

Obesity can cause many health conditions, including hypertension, diabetes, chronic pain, arthritis, and more. Excess weight also contributes to varying levels of inflammation. Studies have shown that obesity does disrupt the immune function in the body. Obesity is known to alter leucocyte, or white blood cell counts, which can affect the immune system. Obesity and inflammation can lead to health complications that affect all areas of the body, including the organs, joints, and bones.[80]

Diet

Diet plays an important part in overall health. A diet that consists of highly processed foods, fried foods, and foods with a lot of sugar and salt will have a negative impact on your immune system and overall health. It is important to do the best you can to eat foods that are healthy. The best options are fresh fruits and vegetables and lean meats. When we opt for foods that don't have the proper amounts of vitamins and minerals, it can reduce the production of antibodies in the immune cells. This can cause a weakened immune system.

---

80 Fátima Pérez de Heredia, Sonia Gómez-Martínez and Ascensión Marcos, "Obesity, Inflammation and the Immune System," *Proceedings of the Nutrition Society* 71, no. 2 (2012): 332–338, doi:10.1017/s0029665112000092.

Stress

Stress can lead to a host of health issues. When we are stressed, we develop unhealthy habits that can also lead to more health complications. Stress is known to cause a weakened immune system. When the body is stressed, it is known to suppress the immune response and block it from functioning properly. Stress causes the body to produce the hormone cortisol. When cortisone levels are high, it can cause weight gain, hypertension, and internal stress on the organs.

It is important to find activities that will help you reduce stress. Eating healthy, exercising, meditation, yoga, and activities that you enjoy can help you decrease stress and feel a sense of peace and calm.

Lack of Sleep

When we were younger, a nap was essential for our growth, rest, and development. As adults, we still need adequate amounts of sleep. Probably not as much as children, but a good seven to eight hours of sleep will do wonders for our health.

During sleep, our bodies naturally heal themselves. This is important for overall function. Sleep also helps our cognitive function and stress levels. Lack of sleep can lead to a disrupted metabolism, impaired judgment, moodiness, and the reduction of proper function of the immune system.

As the body heals during sleep, there are certain proteins that help the immune system. Cytokines are a protein that is only released during sleep. This protein aids the reduction of inflammation and infection in the body. In addition, while the body is asleep it also produces T-cells. Many of us may wish we had the opportunity to nap like we did when we were kids. Although that may not be an option for some of us, you can still try to commit to getting enough sleep so your body can heal and stay healthy.

Aging

Aging is a natural process in life that comes with many wonderful gifts. What we do while we are young can have an impact during our later years. Even as we do our part to stay as healthy as possible, there are many changes in our bodies that happen as we age, depending on our overall health condition. This includes weakened bones, thinner skin, weakened muscle mass, and more.

As we age, we have to pay closer attention to our health. In general, with aging, the internal organs are not as strong and as a result, the immune cells are not produced as rapidly and effectively. Another thing that can happen is vitamin and mineral deficiencies, specifically micronutrient deficiencies. This can also lead to a weakened immune system. Some health conditions such as Parkinson's disease, osteoarthritis, and heart disease can reduce the proper function of the immune system due to its inflammatory nature and common aging. When the immune system is not working properly, this can cause additional illness and some complications.

Allergies

Substances such as pollen, mold, and/or certain foods can cause an allergic reaction. When a person is allergic to a substance, the body will overact, and the immune system will start to fully attack the substance. As the immune system gets ready to attack the substance, there are times when the immune system is attacking the allergen as if it were a pathogen. There are medications that help individuals with allergies.

Autoimmune Disease

When people have autoimmune diseases, the immune system releases autoantibodies, immune proteins that are known to attack organs and tissues. The area that is affected by the immune system is dependent on the specific autoimmune condition. The immune system mistakes the affected part of the body, skin, and/or joints from the autoimmune disease as a foreign and threatening object. Some autoimmune diseases include conditions such as diabetes, lupus, arthritis, inflammatory bowel disease, Multiple Sclerosis, Graves' disease, rheumatoid arthritis, psoriasis, and Hashimoto's disease.

Illnesses

A number of illnesses can affect the immune system and result in a greater chance of getting sick more often. Some of the illnesses include lymphoma, leukemia, HIV, myeloma, sepsis, monoecious, and some cancers.

Medication

Some health conditions require long-term medication. Some side effects of medications are known to weaken the immune system. Sometimes this can create a worse outcome because the condition itself may already lead to a weakened immune system. Some of the medications that are known to weaken the immune system include treatments for arthritis, organ transplants, lupus, IBS, allergies, chemotherapy, and corticosteroids.

CHAPTER TEN

Brain Function and Copper

Brain health is important for the overall function of the body. Staying active with exercise, getting proper sleep, and staying hydrated are general ways to keep the brain healthy. Engaging in regular activities that promote active use of the brain is beneficial for not only our brain health but our overall health and lifestyle.

Some activities that can help the health of the brain include reading, playing a musical instrument, physical activity, puzzles, and art. Having an active social life can also help with brain health as it reduces the symptoms of isolation and loneliness. Nutrition is also an important part of brain health. Eating a well-balanced diet with an abundance of fruits and vegetables will also help to keep both the body and brain healthy.

Vitamins and minerals also play an important role. Copper is a very important factor when it comes to the development and health of the brain.

Copper is an important mineral that supports brain function.

If a person has too much copper, it can negatively affect the brain. Too much copper in the brain can result in the reduction of dopamine levels and the increase of mental health conditions such as depression. If a person doesn't have enough copper in the body, it can also negatively affect the brain, so balance is key.

It is also important that copper, along with other vitamins and minerals, is properly absorbed. The brain has a natural function that can regulate the copper metabolism in the organ. For example, astrocytes, which are the white matter in the brain, are known to regulate the copper that is in the brain.

If there is not enough copper in the body and the regulation of the copper is deficient, this can cause neurodegeneration disorders. Some of the conditions include the following:

Huntington's disease—This is a genetic disorder that causes personality changes, memory issues, and chorea or involuntary body movements.

Menkes disease—This is a condition that is genetic and occurs when the ATP7A gene doesn't work properly in the body. This is discussed on page 51.

Parkinson's disease—This is a disease that affects the nervous system due to the loss of neurons in the brain.

Occipital horn syndrome—This is a condition that is genetic and caused by changes in the ATP7A gene and that affects the skeletal, nervous system, and connective tissue.[81]

---

81 Svetlana Lutsenko et al., "Copper and the Brain Noradrenergic System," *JBIC Journal of Biological Inorganic Chemistry* 24, no. 8 (2019): 1179–1188, doi:10.1007/s00775-019-01737-3.

Wilson's disease—This is a disease where the body is not able to remove extra copper in the body on its own.

Although this is not the leading factor for some of these diseases, copper does play a strong role in overall brain function and development.

This chapter will explore the anatomy of the brain, some ways that you can keep the brain healthy, and the way copper can impact brain function.

The Anatomy of the Brain

The brain is known as one of the most complex organs in the body. It is the organ that controls the processes that regulate many areas of our body. This includes but is not limited to our thought process, memory, touch, vision, breathing, motor skills, and temperature. An adult brain weighs approximately 3 pounds. The makeup of the brain is a combination of water, fat, protein, carbohydrates, and salts. The brain also has nerves and blood vessels.

The brain and the spinal cord make up part of the central nervous system. The central nervous system has two different regions. They are the gray matter and white matter. The white matter is the inner section of the brain. This portion has axons, the connectors of neurons, and a protective coating called myelin. The gray matter is the outer portion and is made of neuron somas, or round cell bodies.

The gray and white matter of the brain work together and have their own functional purpose. The white matter sends messages to parts of the nervous system while the gray matter interprets and processes the information that is located in the brain. The spinal cord also has gray and white matter. The placement of the gray and white matter is different in the spinal cord. The gray matter is located on the inner portion and the white matter sits on the outer portion of the central nervous system. The spinal cord carries nerve signals from the brain to the body.

We are not really conscious of it, but the brain is actively receiving and sending signals throughout the body. Depending on the signals, the brain will process the messages differently. Some messages are felt throughout the body and some stay within the brain.

The Cerebrum, Cerebellum, and Brainstem

It is important to understand how the brain works and functions in order to understand why and how copper benefits the brain. Copper is essential for the proper function of the brain and it is present in the cerebellum.

The brain has three major parts: the cerebellum (back of the head), cerebrum (front of the brain), and brainstem (bottom of the brain and connects the spinal cord).

The cerebrum is the largest part of the brain. This area of the brain part has both gray matter and white matter. This area of the brain also has two halves, or hemispheres. The right hemisphere of the cerebral cortex controls the operation of the left side of the body. The left side of the cerebral cortex controls the operation of the right side of the body. Together they communicate through a nerve called the corpus callosum, an area of white matter that is located at the center of the cerebrum.

The function of this area of the brain includes thinking, emotions, problem-solving, judgment, speech, vision, hearing, and the senses. This area of the brain also regulates movement and temperature within the body.

The cerebellum is a small portion of the brain that is housed in the back of the head that includes the brainstem and part of the spinal cord. This area of the brain also has two hemispheres: the outer hemisphere and the inner hemisphere. The outer hemisphere has neurons, and the inner hemisphere interacts with the cerebral cortex. This area of the brain helps the body with muscle movements, balance, posture, heart rate, and respiration.

The brainstem is the middle of the brain. It includes three sections: the midbrain (mesenchephalon), the pons, and the medulla. The brainstem connects the cerebrum and the spinal cord. Each area of this section of the brain plays an important role in our body. The mesencephalon has a plethora of neural pathways and clusters. This area of the brain helps the body function in many ways—this includes processing calculations, hearing, movement, and coordination.

The Pons, Medulla, and Spinal Cord

The pons is the area that connects the midbrain and the bottom of the brain stem. The pons is the area of the brain that is responsible for helping the body balance, create facial expressions, chew, blink, see clearly, and produce tears.

The medulla is the area of the brain that helps the body survive. This area of the brain is located at the bottom of the brainstem, where the brain and the spinal cord meet. The medulla activates the area of the brain that causes us to physically breathe, cough, swallow, and vomit. This area of the brain is also known to regulate breathing, oxygen, heart rhythm, and carbon dioxide.

The spinal cord is located in the bottom of the skull. Extending from the bottom of the medulla, this area is responsible for communicating messages from the brain to the body.

The Protective Covering of the Brain

Along with the areas of the brain, the organ also has a protective covering. This area is called the meninges. It surrounds the spinal cord and the brain. There are three layers of this protective covering: the pia, arachnoid mater, and the dura mater.

The pia has a thin mater that supports the surface and contours of the brain. There is a collection of web-like connective tissue called the arachnoid, and the cerebrospinal fluid of the brain is housed under the arachnoid. This part of the protective covering is important because it creates a soft safety net for the full nervous system. It also protects the area from bacteria by removing impurities and other unnecessary fluids.

The arachnoid mater is a thin middle layer that is housed between the pia mater and dura mater. This area has fluid that cushions the brain and doesn't have nerves or blood vessels.

The dura mater is the outermost layer. This area has two layers that line the area of the skull. This area supports the movement of the arteries and veins that supply necessary blood flow to the brain.

There are also four different lobes that are responsible for proper brain function. The frontal lobe is the largest and sits at the front of the head. This area helps the body with its decision-making abilities. It is also the area that aids in forming personality, speech ability, and the recognition of aromas and smells. The parietal lobe is in the middle of the brain. This is the area that recognizes touch, pain, and special relationships. This area also helps the brain process and understand spoken language. The occipital lobe helps with vision and the temporal lobe helps the brain with speech, rhythm, music, and short-term memory. Along with the rest of the anatomy of the brain, collectively everything works together to keep the brain functioning properly so it can send signals to the body to do the same. This is one of the many reasons why brain health is important.[82]

Keeping the Brain Healthy

Just like the body, there are a number of ways that you can keep your brain healthy. One way that you've read many times in this book is with proper nutrition, exercise, and maintaining a healthy and active lifestyle. The brain is so intricate it affects the whole body. We may not give our brains much thought. It shows up for us daily in different ways. We can do our part to keep it as healthy as possible.

The health of the brain also is a determinant of how different areas of the mind and body function. There are different areas of the brain that are responsible for the different functions and how we react. For example, the tactile function determines how you respond to pressure, temperature, and pain. The emotional function shows how you respond to emotions, the motor func-

---

82 "Brain Anatomy and How the Brain Works," John Hopkins Medicine, accessed August 30, 2022, https://www.hopkinsmedicine.org/health /conditions-and-diseases/anatomy-of-the-brain.

tion shows the ability to control movements and balance. The cognitive function determines thinking, memory, and learning.

These are general categories. There are many factors as to why people move, react, and respond to pain. Brain health can be affected by many factors. This includes but is not limited to stress, changes in the brain due to age, injuries that affect the brain, stroke, heart conditions, addiction, depression, substance abuse, and/or mood disorders. In addition, other factors include diseases that affect the brain and the neurological system. Brain health is not one size fits all.

Here are some general tips and suggested lifestyle habits that can help the brain stay healthy. If you do have a health condition that affects the brain, have a discussion with your doctor regarding a plan to help your health condition, brain, and overall health.

Eating Healthy

It is important to eat a diet that is rich in essential vitamins and minerals. Reducing the intake of processed foods, fried foods, sugar, salt, alcohol, and nicotine can play a large part in your overall health as well as the function of the brain. There are some specific foods that are known to help the overall health of your brain.

- Avocado
- Banana
- Broccoli
- Chamomile tea
- Chia seeds
- Cod
- Collards
- Eggs
- Green tea
- Kale

- Lentils
- Matcha tea
- Pollack
- Quinoa

- Salmon
- Walnuts
- Water

The brain foods that have copper are avocado, chia seeds, quinoa, and salmon. All of the listed foods and beverages have benefits that also help other areas of the body along with the brain. There are many ways that you can incorporate these foods into your diet.

Exercise

It is important to exercise your body and brain by staying active. When you exercise it will increase your mood, help with your mobility and balance, strengthen bones, help you maintain a healthy weight, help the strength and flexibility of the muscles, and also help your mind and brain function.

Exercise also increases your energy, reduces inflammation, reduces stress, and aids in keeping stress hormones low. Regular exercise also aids in helping heart health and cholesterol levels and is known to reduce the symptoms of diabetes.

A regular habit of exercise can also aid in the prevention of illnesses such as heart disease, diabetes, and some neurological disorders. There are a lot of ways to incorporate exercise into your daily schedule You can walk, jog, swim, or practice yoga, tai chi, or Pilates just to name a few. For the older population who may not be as mobile, there are many options such as chair exercises and activites that are age-appropriate for physical development and mobility. Don't underestimate the many ways we naturally move throughout the day. This can include running errands, shopping, moving around at the office, and even moving around at home. Simple household chores are a form of mild exercise and movement. From vacuuming to dusting to wiping items, and for those who clean with music, dancing. Exercise can improve the function of the brain in several ways.

A regular habit of exercise and physical activity can help the function of the brain. When we exercise, there are some hormones that are released that aid in brain function.

As the body is in movement through exercise, neurotransmitters are released. These are chemical signals that send messages throughout the nervous system. Along with the neurotransmitters, some of the hormones that are released due to exercise are endorphins. These are the hormones that increase the feeling of pleasure. Another hormone is endocannabinoids, which give the feeling of calmness and excitement—this hormone is described to give the feeling of the runners high. This is helpful for the brain because it brings clarity, and motivation, and increases mood.[83]

Another hormone that is actively activated by exercise is dopamine. This hormone is known to aid in helping the body with increasing focus, learning, and concentration; stabilizing the mood; and increasing motivation. It also regulates the heart rate and helps the body rest by aiding in regulating better sleep patterns. This is helpful because during sleep the body has an opportunity to support the brain by helping it detox and cleanse

83 "Cognitive Health and Older Adults," National Institute on Aging, October 1, 2020, https://www.nia.nih.gov/health/cognitive-health-and-older-adults.

waste from the central nervous system. Sleep helps reduce stress. Proper sleep can also help the cognitive function of the body.[84]

Studies have shown that regular physical activity can help delay the aging process of the brain and reverse some of the complications that come from a sedentary lifestyle. Engaging in a habit of regular exercise is also known to help reduce some symptoms of neurological disorders and degenerative diseases.[85]

A habit of regular exercise can do wonders for the body. For beginners start with 10 minutes a day three times a day to make your 30 minutes and gradually move up from there. Find activities that you truly enjoy so you will stay consistent. If you already have a habit of exercise incorporated in your lifestyle, continue to maintain your health.

Reduce Stress

Stress can impact health in many ways that we may not even realize. When we are stressed, our internal organs are strongly impacted, and this includes the brain. Studies have shown that stress has the ability to shrink the brain, disrupt memory, and kill brain cells in the brain's hippocampus. This is one of the areas where new brain cells are formed. The hippocampus is also the area that impacts learning, memory, and emotion. Stress can

---

84 Julia C. Basso and Wendy A. Suzuki, "The Effects of Acute Exercise on Mood, Cognition, Neurophysiology, and Neurochemical Pathways: A Review," *Brain Plasticity* 2, no. 2 (2017): 127–152, doi:10.3233/bpl-160040.

85 Di Liegro et al., "Physical Activity and Brain Health," *Genes* 10, no. 9 (2019): 720, doi:10.3390/genes10090720.

also increase the risk of health conditions such as obesity, stroke, heart-related illness, and diabetes.[86]

When we are stressed, sometimes we don't realize it and we react in a way that is not our behavioral norm. This can cause overeating, overindulging, and at times depression and anxiety. Other symptoms of stress include the following:

o Digestive issues

o Exhaustion

o Insomnia

o Irritability

o Low libido

o Pain in different areas of the body

o Rapid heartbeat

o Sadness

o Weakened immune system

o Weight gain

One of the best ways to identify and reduce stress is to know yourself and your body. There are times when we are busy, tired, and moving in many different directions. We adapt and allow this to become the norm. The tasks keep piling on without our realizing it, we don't allow ourselves to take a break, and we just keep going. In the meantime, stress is building in our bodies. Long-term stress can lead to illness.

Learn to pause and check in with yourself. First, check your breathing. If it is short and you are breathing from the upper area of the chest, pause and give yourself some full breaths to nourish the body. Check in with yourself to see how you respond to regular tasks. If you are easily annoyed or feel overwhelmed about doing a mundane task, this could indicate a high level

---

86 R. M. Thomas, G. Hotsenpiller and D. A. Peterson, "Acute Psychosocial Stress Reduces Cell Survival in Adult Hippocampal Neurogenesis Without Altering Proliferation," *Journal of Neuroscience* 27, no. 11 (2007): 2734–2743, doi:10.1523/jneurosci.3849-06.2007.

of stress or exhaustion. It is important to pause and take time to reduce stress in your life. This is important for your overall health. Here are some activities that you can engage in that will help you reduce stress.

o Breathing exercises   o Sleep

o Eating a healthy diet   o Self-care

o Gratitude practice   o Taking a break

o Journaling   o Therapy

o Meditation   o Yoga

o Physical activity

Social Interaction

Engaging in the world around you and maintaining healthy relationships with family and friends can help reduce the feeling of isolation and loneliness. This helps your brain by engaging with different people and activities. There are many things you can do to keep a healthy social life. Spend time with friends, volunteer, take a class, work toward a cause that you are passionate about, teach on a subject that you know about, join social clubs that are focused on topics that interest you, and enjoy social outings and events.

There are many ways to keep the brain active and healthy. There are some vitamins and minerals that also help the health of the brain and this includes copper.

Copper and the Brain

Copper is an important mineral to have for overall brain function. Proper copper levels can help reduce some brain-related illnesses. Copper helps proper brain function because the demand for oxygen in the brain is highly dependent on copper. A copper deficiency can negatively affect brain function, as can an excess amount of copper. It is important to keep the proper levels of copper in the body so it can be regulated throughout the brain and body to keep it healthy.[87]

With such a central role in the brain, copper also affects a gene in the body called ATP7A. This is a gene that aids in making a protein that is key in regulating copper levels in the body. It is housed in the Golgi apparatus, a cell structure in the body. Inside the Golgi apparatus, the ATP7A protein helps to sustain healthy copper levels in the body.

It does this by feeding copper to specific enzymes that are responsible for the function, structure, and growth of the blood vessels, hair, skin, bones, and nervous system.[88]

The ATP7A gene has its place in and throughout the body. It is housed in a cell structure called the Golgi apparatus. This is the area in the body that structures enzymes and new proteins that are produced in the body. It is spread everywhere except in the liver cells.

87 Ivo F. Scheiber, Julian F.B. Mercer and Ralf Dringen, "Metabolism and Functions of Copper in Brain," *Progress in Neurobiology* 116 (2014): 33–57, doi:10.1016/j.pneurobio.2014.01.002.

88 Stephen G. Kaler, "ATP7A-Related Copper Transport Diseases—Emerging Concepts and Future Trends," *Nature Reviews Neurology* 7, no. 1 (2011): 15–29, doi:10.1038/nrneurol.2010.180.

Although this gene is one of the helpers to regulate copper levels in the body and help neurological function, if there is a defect in ATP7A, it can cause Menkes disease. As mentioned, this is a health condition that affects the physical and mental development of the body. This condition happens when the body can't properly absorb and transport copper throughout the body. When this happens, this causes problems with the blood vessels, nerve function, intellectual ability, and the development of the structure of the hair, skin, and bones. Children with this dysfunction are known to have seizures and mental dysfunction.

This disease is typically inherited and in some cases, it is not. This condition is primarily developed during infancy, though there are some situations where it is developed later in childhood, but this is rare. Copper is known to help some of the symptoms of this disease.[89]

Some of the many areas where copper is present in the brain is the hippocampus, basal ganglia, cerebellum, synaptic membranes, and cerebellar granular neurons. Along with having an impact in these areas, there are also some enzymes that are located in the central nervous system that need copper to function properly. Some of these enzymes include peptidyl glycine, tyrosinase, hephaestin, copper/zinc superoxide dismutase, hephaestin, peptidyl glycine α-amidating mono-oxygenase, dopamine-β-hydroxylase, and cytochrome c oxidase.

Copper is noted as an impactful cofactor or helper to assist enzymes in carrying functions that they can't do on their own such as the healthy and proper function of the neurological

---

89 Svetlana Lutsenko et al., "Copper and the Brain Noradrenergic System," *JBIC Journal of Biological Inorganic Chemistry* 24, no. 8 (2019): 1179–1188, doi:10.1007/s00775-019-01737-3.

system. Although copper is a mineral that is needed for healthy body function, it also needs to be regulated due to its potentially harmful effects on the body if it is not excreted effectively and properly.

CHAPTER ELEVEN

Copper and Energy Levels

Energy in the body is typically delivered through the food and drinks that we consume. This is why it is important to eat healthy, nutrient-infused foods and avoid processed foods with a lot of salt and sugar. It is the metabolism that changes the food we consume into energy. The primary nutrients that give our bodies energy from food are healthy fats, protein, and carbohydrates. Each of these nutrients can pull from each other to give the body the energy that it needs.

Other ways to get energy are staying hydrated with water, proper rest, and keeping stress levels low. There are some foods that can give the body higher levels of energy, such as bananas, salmon, tuna, berries, and oats. Collectively these foods have vitamins and minerals such as vitamin B6, antioxidants, fiber, carbs, and protein. Another mineral that helps the body with minerals is copper.

Copper is a cofactor of many enzymes that helps produce energy throughout the body. Other benefits of copper include, but are not limited to, metabolizing iron in the body, helping energy production, and keeping the blood vessels healthy. This will help energy levels and vitality.[90]

Energy and Copper

There is nothing like having consistent energy to accomplish the things that we have to do and have extra energy to enjoy activities that we want to do. In a perfect world, we have energy when we need it and when we don't. There are specific times of day when we feel tired and there are times when fatigue takes over from throughout the whole day. The level of tiredness is circumstantial depending on your lifestyle and schedule

For adults, and for some children and adolescents, schedules can be full, with rest being an afterthought. Some people are consistently fatigued and feel as if their energy is completely depleted. This can come from a variety of reasons, such as illness, stress, a busy schedule, lack of proper nutrition, poor diet, some medications, disrupted sleep patterns, and/or a vitamin deficiency. There are different ways to increase your energy so you can feel like you can get through your day and beyond. This chapter discusses how energy is formed in the body, the different ways to sustain energy levels, and the ways that copper affects energy levels in the body.

90 Svetlana Lutsenko, "Human Copper Homeostasis: A Network of Interconnected Pathways," *Current Opinion in Chemical Biology* 14, no. 2 (2010): 211–217, doi:10.1016/j.cbpa.2010.01.003.

Energy in the Body

In the human body, energy comes from fuel molecules. These molecules consist of carbohydrates, lipids, and proteins. Once the molecules are in the body, these energy levels are then shifted into other chemical forms of energy that the body needs to function properly.

When we consume food, the body can convert it to energy. There is a chemical energy called adenosine triphosphate (ATP). The energy from this chemical comes from broken-down food molecules. These molecules then release energy to other cellular processes like metabolism, protein synthesis, and cellular respiration. Although there are small amounts of ATP that are stored in the body, this chemical energy needs to be generated on a continuous basis so it can function properly.

The way to generate this energy is through food. Typically, food consists of vitamins, minerals, and other nutritional agents. Some include proteins, fats, and carbohydrates. When the food is consumed it is broken down into amino acids, glucose, and fatty acids. Each of these compounds is utilized or stored. Fats are typically used for long-term energy, and carbohydrates are typically used for short-term energy needs. Proteins help the body build muscles.

There are three energy systems that give the cells ATP so they can function properly in the body. Although they are three different energy systems, they work together so the body has proper energy levels. The systems are the following.

The Aerobic Oxidative System

The aerobic oxidative system breaks down and processes the nutrients in the body. This system gives the majority of the body's ATP. This energy system is used when the body is in physical movement. It can fuel the body with ATP for longer periods of time.

When you are moving your body and energy is needed, this system supplies nutrients to the body. These nutrients include glucose, carbohydrates, fatty acids, and proteins. Generally, the body will use fatty acids to supply energy. When the body is in need of more energy due to more physical movement or if a person is participating in exercise, carbohydrates are used to give the body the energy that it needs. Protein is also used to supply energy, but it is not a major source. For the aerobic oxidative system to generate ATP, oxygen is needed from the respiratory and cardiovascular systems. Although the aerobic oxidative system provides energy from physical movement, it also helps the body repair and builds tissues, controls its temperature, digest food, and helps with hair growth.

The Anaerobic System

The anaerobic system, also called the lactic acid system, doesn't require oxygen. With this system, glycolysis produces energy that is needed and breaks down into glucose. This occurs when there are short and intense levels of energy needed. For example, if a person is running sprints or adding momentum to an exercise, the lactic acid levels will rise and fuel the body for short periods of time. When the body is undergoing intense exercise and there is an accumulation of lactic acid, the feeling of a burning sensation and tiredness in the muscles will occur.

The Phosphagen Energy System

The phosphagen energy system is also called the ATP-CP system. This system uses creatine phosphate (CP). This is stored in the muscle cells to rapidly produce ATP. This system doesn't use oxygen because it is anaerobic. The phosphagen energy system is activated when a person starts an activity. This energy source is used during the initial seconds. It is also used during short and intense sessions of physical activity. When the ATP is released and depleted from the intensity of the movements in the body, the body will produce more ATP by breaking down creatine phosphate that is stored in the muscles and fueling itself with energy. Copper helps with cellular energy production.

When we think of the energy system in the body and how it works together to give us the energy that we need, think of it in levels. The aerobic energy system produces energy for the movements of the body that are low intensity, long duration, and/or endurance. The anaerobic system supplies energy to movements that are medium to high intensity. Finally, the phosphagen energy system (ATP-CP) supports high-intensity movements that may come in the form of short bursts of time.

Increase Energy Levels

There are several ways to increase your energy. Three of the main ways are with exercise, eating properly (see page 75), and hydration. These three areas are actionable items that you can incorporate into your lifestyle.

Exercise

Regular exercise is a wonderful way to maintain good health. A regular habit of physical activity gives the body many benefits. This includes but is not limited to a better mood, reducing the potential of being diagnosed with a health condition, enhanced immunity, increased flexibility and mobility, and an improved ability to focus and concentrate. Exercise can also increase energy, reduce the feeling of tiredness and fatigue, and improve sleep. A regular habit of physical activity will help your body and mind in many ways. Find an activity that you enjoy, gather some friends, or find a class and move your body. It will help you both short and long-term. [91]

Keep Your Body Hydrated

It is important to stay hydrated and drink enough water throughout the day. Even if you consume a lot of beverages, they may not give the proper hydration that is necessary to keep the body healthy. For example, energy drinks, sports drinks, fruit juice, and carbonated drinks have more sugar and empty calories. Getting the proper amounts of water can do wonders for the body. There are some people who don't love the taste of plain water. You can add fresh fruits to give the water some additional flavor; this will also provide additional nutrients from the fruits and vegetables. You can add lemon, cucumber, mint, lime, rasp-

---

91 Gregory N. Ruegsegger and Frank W. Booth, "Health Benefits of Exercise," *Cold Spring Harbor Perspectives in Medicine* 8, no. 7 (2017): a029694, doi:10.1101/cshperspect.a029694.

berries, watermelon, and/or a combination of produce. A strawberry-lime-infused water or a strawberry-lemon combo works well. Mint and lemon are also a good combination.

Dehydration is known to have an effect on your energy levels, brain function, mobility, and mood. When the body is hydrated and consuming the proper amounts of water, it is known to help immune health by preventing infections, serving as a natural detox and filtration system, decreasing joint pain, and aiding in proper organ functioning while delivering nutrients to the cells. Collectively this can help your energy levels.[92]

There are some habits that may be taking a toll on your energy levels. These include too much screen time, scrolling on social media, straining the eyes, consuming too little vitamins and/or minerals, consistently eating on the go, consuming excessive alcohol, smoking, disrupting your sleep cycles, failing to address stress, or taking certain types of medication.

Energy levels vary in everyone. Vitamins and minerals play a part in our energy consumption and function. Copper is a key mineral that helps in energy production.

92 Kory Taylor and Elizabeth Jones, "Adult Dehydration," John Hopkins Medicine, May 15, 2022, https://www.ncbi.nlm.nih.gov/books/NBK555956.

Conclusion: Copper and Your Health Journey

As you read through the pages of this book, you learned a lot about the health and healing benefits that copper offers. You also learned there are a lot of ways that copper plays an important role in our daily lives. Copper is a metal that is multifaceted and impacts us more than we realize.

The focus of this book was on health and healing, and I encourage you to reflect on your own health and healing journey. Remember it is not one size fits all nor is it a straight line. We are human beings that are consistently growing, learning, and hopefully, working toward becoming the best versions of ourselves.

Copper has an important role to play in our bodies. There are many ways that you can consume copper through many delicious food options. You can also take a supplement. Just like copper, there are many vitamins and minerals that are essential for our overall health. It is best if you can consume your vitamins and minerals through food. If you need a supplement, that is perfectly fine as well.

There are a lot of wonderful ways that you can incorporate these foods into your diet. There are also a lot of recipes that you can create. Enjoy the process and also know by consuming these foods, you are also getting additional vitamins, minerals, and health benefits.

See the list of copper-enriched foods on page 77.

As you start or continue your health journey, remember to look at your life from a holistic perspective and focus on each area as needed. This is your journey and the beauty of it is to see how much you've grown along the way. It takes a lot of courage to change your life. Making the decision and following through is a wonderful accomplishment. Don't forget to enjoy the process and celebrate yourself along the way.

All change takes time. Give yourself the space you need to gently move into the new version of yourself. Remember to try to do something consistently that your future self will thank you for. It doesn't have to be all at one time. Small, consistent steps can lead to big and impactful results. Take it one day at a time and be intentional about your thoughts, actions, and words.

Your health journey is yours. As you work on your goals, grow through them, and move on to the next, it is important to consistently learn about ways to improve your health and overall life. Reading is one of them. Take your time to learn the information that you come across. Incorporate the information in your life as you see fit. Sometimes we learn information that can be used instantly or later down the line. For some, it is weeks, months, or years. Either way, you now have the knowledge. You can pass it along and share it with others who may benefit.

As you start or continue your health journey, may you find the patience, strength, courage, and determination to continue. Give yourself grace, love, and compassion. This is your life, and you deserve to live a life that you love.

Acknowledgments

I give thanks and the highest praise to God for orchestrating this opportunity and showing me the way to live my life purpose and dreams.

Thank you to my friends, family, community, and supporters. Thank you for your support, words of encouragement, con-sis-tent prayers, and love. I am deeply grateful for each of you. Thank you for creating space for technicolor dreams, pure bliss, and endless memories. Thank you for seeing my light when I was blinded by darkness and hearing my screams through silence. This has been a long journey with a long way to go. Thank you for riding this crazy, blissful, creative ride with me.

Thank you to my writing community and those who were and still are a part of my writing journey.

Thank you to the team at Ulysses Press and Simon & Schuster. I am deeply grateful for your patience, guidance, and support.

Thank you to our literacy ancestors who persisted with leaving records of their genius even when their genius wasn't allowed, celebrated, or recognized. To those who take up the mantle in honor of our literary ancestors and their work, remember that this is a continuum. May you keep the faith to make your dreams come true and be a light for others passing the torch now and forever.

Yves Stines, Bettye Stines, Bettina Ortez, Joshua Ortez, Raymonde Stines, Dr. Linda Nabha, Charlena Ponders, Eliza-beth Whittaker-Walker, Dr. LeConte Dill, Casie Vogel, Shelona Belfon, Kinyel Friday, Jason Johns, Francina James, Julie D. Andrews, Jonathan Schwartz, Roderica James, Cely Maria Dias, Keith Goldstein, Terrance Smith, Kerri Johnson, April Ray, Derek Hunter, Rebecca Rudnicki, Aaron Seller, Rae Chesny, Nikki Johnson, Deidre Bounds, Nikki Pardo, Aimee DuFresne, Victoria C. Rowan, Louise Spector, and Arnold Hamilton – thank you.

If you made it to this page, thank you for reading my book. May you find the courage, peace, and freedom to live a healthy life that you love. God bless you!

About the Author

Yvelette Stines is a writer, teacher, and storyteller whose work educates, entertains, and creates safe spaces for individuals to evolve, flourish, and mature, holistically. Stines's work reaches a broad audience, and has been featured in renowned publications including Essence, Business Insider, SHAPE, T Brand Studio of The New York Times, Mind Body Green, Healthline, The Source, and more. She is a thought leader and an accomplished author of six books and journals related to lifestyle, health, and wellness.

As a writer, Stines leverages her invaluable experience in both education and public relations to develop messaging that resonates with multiple generations. Understanding that her audience lived dynamic and unique experiences, she taps into her teaching background to lead them to translate intentions into action, driving them closer to the life that they want. Her workshops take participants through a journey of self-discovery to achieving meaningful mind, body, and soul change, without compromising their values and priorities.

In addition to guiding individuals to become better versions of themselves, Stines amplifies her impact by advancing equity in health and wellness. She has developed well-received programs for women and children encouraging them to create and sustain wellness practices that inspire and motivate them to achieve an intentional and well-rounded lifestyle.

Stines prides herself on practicing what she preaches. She is continuously evolving, growing, and pivoting as more of her life's purpose reveals itself. While living out her purpose and creating her legacy through writing, wellness, and teaching, Stines finds balance in enjoying other leisure activities including traveling, photography, exploring culinary arts, and spending time outdoors. She continues to live life with an aligned purpose and encourages others to do the same.

Website: www.yvelettestines.com